MANAGIN

HEALTH SERVICES

MANAGING COMMUNITY HEALTH SERVICES

Edited by
Allan McNaught

CHAPMAN AND HALL

LONDON · NEW YORK · TOKYO · MELBOURNE · MADRAS

UK   Chapman and Hall, 2–6 Boundary Row, London SE1 8HN

USA   Chapman and Hall, 29 West 35th Street, New York NY10001

JAPAN   Chapman and Hall Japan, Thomson Publishing Japan,
            Hirakawacho Nemoto Building, 7F, 1–7–11 Hirakawa-cho,
            Chiyoda-ku, Tokyo 102

AUSTRALIA   Chapman and Hall Australia, Thomas Nelson Australia, 102
            Dodds Street, South Melbourne, Victoria 3205

INDIA   Chapman and Hall India, R. Seshadri, 32 Second Main Road,
            CIT East, Madras 600 035

First edition 1991

© 1991 Allan McNaught

Phototypeset in 10/12 Souvenir Light by
Input Typesetting Ltd, London
Printed in Great Britain by
St Edmundsbury Press, Bury St Edmunds, Suffolk

ISBN 0 412 31900 4

British Library Cataloguing in Publication Data

Managing community health services.
  1. Great Britain. Community health services
  I. McNaught, Allan, *1952–*
  362.10425

  ISBN 0 412 31900 4

Library of Congress Cataloging-in-Publication Data

available

Contents

Contributors

Gillian Dalley was a Research Fellow at the Centre for Health Economics, University of York, she is now a Research Fellow with the Policy Studies Institute, London.

Robin Douglas is Head of Management Education and Development with the Office for Public Management. He was previously a Faculty Member of the King's Fund College.

Rosemary Dun is currently combining the full-time care of her first child with writing on health policy and other issues. Her past employment has included work in rehabilitation in the NHS and in the voluntary sector around issues of disability and care in the community. More recently she was employed by West Lambeth Health Authority to explore the practical applications of patch-based primary health care and community health services.

Jenny Harrow is a Principal Lecturer in the Centre for Management Studies at Southbank Polytechnic. She is Course Director for the part-time MSC Public Service Management.

Su Kingsley was formerly a Faculty member of the King's Fund College. She is now Director of Corporate Planning with Lambeth, Southwark and Lewisham Family Health Services Authority.

Margaret McArthur now works for South West Surrey Health Authority as Contracts Development Manager. She was previously a Management Associate with the Management Advisory Service to the NHS.

Allan McNaught is Director of Planning and Service Development with the Merton, Sutton and Wandsworth Family Health Services Authority. Previously, he was Programme Director: Health Administration, with the Overseas Development Administration, London, and was on loan to the Government of Zimbabwe for two years.

Simon Stone was a Management Associate with the Management Advisory Service to the NHS. Simon is now the Director of Nursing at Kidderminster General Hospital.

Glenn Warren is Unit General Manager–Community with North Staffordshire Health Authority.

Editor's introduction

This book was originally conceived in 1987. It was then seen as a contribution towards improved management and policy-making in a diffuse and neglected area of NHS management. The focus of the book is the 'old' Community Health Services: those transferred to Area Health Authorities from local authorities in the 1974 re-organization of the NHS. These diverse services, while grouped together, had little objectively in common, occupying, as they do, a hazy middle ground between hospital and Family Practitioner Services.

However, since 1974 there have been a number of major developments which have opened opportunities for change and development in these services. These include: the resurrection of concern with 'Public Health'; the attempted closure of large mental illness and mental handicap hospitals and the development of 'Community Care'; the introduction of General Management; and the implication for health and local authorities of the White Papers 'Caring for People', 'Promoting Better Health' and 'Working for Patients'.

Traditionally, Community Health Services were seen as low status and a professional dead-end. This, in turn, has led to a rather uneven body of literature. The growth of general management has led to a demand for a more coherent, management-orientated literature. It is our hope that this book will encourage the production of more literature in this area.

The development of Community Care offers some interesting parallels and lessons. The attempt to provide long-term care on a community basis has demonstrated some of the enormous difficulties, philosophical and practical, of providing any service on an integrated basis in the community. The problems involved with working with local authorities, voluntary agencies, as well as other parts of the NHS, are not always self evident, or surmountable.

Managing Community Health Services does not see its mission as providing managers and policy makers with 'off the shelf' answers, even if these were possible to provide. The problems in this area of health and social care are formidable, and there is a very wide range of actors and providers in the policy arena. The lead role being given to local authorities by 'Caring for People' and the emphasis on purchasing services does little to change the dynamics here, although it does mean fairly fundamental procedural and cultural change.

While not offering ready answers, this book will try to explore some of the constraints, challenges and the context of this rapidly changing policy and management framework, and try to bring some key problems into clearer relief.

Finally, this book is not exactly as planned in 1987. Several valuable contributors have had to drop out, and much of the editing was done at long distance, while I was on contract in Zimbabwe. However, many thanks to Christine and Terri at Chapman and Hall, who did a great deal to keep the project on the road, and to the final contributors who stuck with the venture.

Allan McNaught
London

Part One

Policy and Management Issues

1

Local authority health strategies

Jenny Harrow

This chapter reviewing the local authority contribution to the 'national health' is in itself symbolic of the changes which have occurred in the health policy environment in Britain. At the level of service delivery, local authority action is also a reaction to a situation in which current community-based health initiatives represent a patchwork of provision, including many examples of experimentation, but with areas left uncovered. Some current thinking on the nature of central/local relations still seems to be tending towards the notion of local government as the agent of central government; for example, Chandler's assessment that most national political actors seek to ensure local government's implementation of policies, determined centrally, to suit local circumstances (Chandler, 1988). This model does not, however, fit easily with a number of examples of local authorities' developing seemingly high profile health strategies. This might be interpreted as a means of making public statements about the value and credibility of local government as such, and as evidence of a local government concern for public well-being which goes well beyond a narrow focus on statutorily-defined duties.

Critics of these developments may see in them local authorities 'searching for a role'. Others may regard elements in some such developments as reflecting, and being motivated by, opposition politics towards central government health policies, as much as any rediscovery of the importance of health issues for the charge-paying public. Useful parallels and contrasts may be made here with the development of local authority unemployment strategies, as discussed by Portwood (1986). Early stages of such work may be characterized by a series of small-scale projects, where major emphases are placed on attitudinal change, followed by a recognition of a need for organizational change; where managerial issues appear to be left to officer groups to resolve, and where liaison and cooperation with other agencies becomes of central importance. An alternative approach is to see the growth of local authorities' health strategies as an inevitable – and essential – outcome of corporate management philosophies, requiring overviews of the environment in which an authority delivers services, and awareness of the impact of the work of other organizations on how it performs. Thus, for example, Slough Borough Council's health strategy statement justifies its development by reference to the degree of interdependence which it sees between service areas, where the omission of health issues would limit the credibility of remaining policy areas:

> . . . without a Health Strategy (which in many respects overlaps some of the objectives in Leisure and Housing), the Council does not have clearly defined objectives to take into account when making policy decisions. (Thomson, undated)

This chapter identifies and discusses examples of developing local authority health strategies impacting upon communities, raising questions as to the continuance of these developments in local authority hands. Undoubtedly the enhanced role for social services departments envisaged by the Griffiths report on community care, and the related likelihood of the continued burgeoning of the voluntary sector to take on service roles for those departments will add urgency to the ways in which local authorities view their involvement – or non-involvement – in health-based issues. The chapter examines the basis of the 'new public health' movement, and the local authority position as reflecting a non-medical model of health concerns; reviews collaborative health strategies with the health service; and considers the development of local authority concern in 'ill health' and the types of objectives and priorities which flow from that. It looks at examples from health strategy documentation; considers the impetus to local authority initiatives, particularly in relation to the creation of health profiles, given by the WHO Healthy Cities programme; and concludes with reference to the government response to the Griffiths report.

The notion of local authorities having 'health strategies' at all may in some senses be seen to conflict with the general thrust of health provision being taken out of the hands of elected members. The proposal in the Health Service White Paper, 'Working for

Patients', that 'local authorities will no longer have a right to appoint members of DHAs' (1989b, p. 65) indicates a clear policy of distancing by the centre of local government from health concerns. The concept of 'strategy', as reviewed by Greenwood (1987) in relation to local government structures, describes an organization adopting an entrepreneurial or proactive stance towards products and change, rather than adopting a defensive 'stay as we are' posture. This suggests a highly developed, maintained and funded series of policies; but in practice these vary in content, style and implementability from authority to authority. For some, the term 'scheme' rather than 'strategy' would seem more appropriate.

Some discussion of the nature of the local authorities' role harks back to a recollection of 'former days' when the publicly valued and respected Medical Officer of Health was a focus for attention on 'public health'. Jacobson (1989) writes:

> There is a sad sentimentality about those who still hanker for the good old days of public health. The old medical officer of health – and his (and it *was* his) local authority health army – would have sorted it all out, some wistfully intone.

Some authorities' health strategy documents commence by emphasis on the loss, in terms of public knowledge, incurred with the abolition of the MOH post, and with it the requirement for that Officer's annual report on the state of health in the community. A 'reinstatement' of this activity, but from a different source, comes, perhaps belatedly, with the Department of Health Circular (88) 64, asking health authorities to assess the state of health of their populations, identify areas for improvement and appoint Directors of Public Health, whose responsibilities include the familiar presentation of an annual report on the local population's health. Although the need for close collaboration with local authorities in this work is recognized, it is clear that central government policy remains that of attempting to keep the major lead for 'public health' within the NHS and thus within the ambit of general management.

Although the regret at the departure of the local authority-based MOH may be widespread, it is also important to note that local authority health concerns are couched in wider terms than those employed by medical professionals, with the possibility at times of challenging medical models of 'health' and 'illness'. Beardshaw assessed that, in 1987, more than a third of urban councils had health committees. She described these bodies as 'fragile . . . still in the process of defining their role', and emphasized that they

> . . . all share an approach to health which centres on its social and economic determinants – housing, nutrition, environmental factors, income – rather than medical ones.

This in turn may suggest that it is in the local authority health field, rather than in the health authority sphere that cross-professional views of community health needs may be voiced strongly, if not lay views, with the direct involvement of elected members.

Whether or not authorities have embarked on publicized health strategies their environmental health services work – refuse collection, pest control, the control of food and drug sales, and the detection and control of health nuisances – has been the basis for local authority health concern. Here, the regulatory and enforcement functions are based statutorily, with minimal public attention until a local or national 'health scare' occurs. Both refuse collection and pest control have been key targets for contracting out to private companies, although in no case does this seem to have been part of a health strategy as such. Developments in environmental health work are, however, limited by staff recruitment and retention problems, particularly in the major conurbations, so that, again, 'schemes' rather than 'strategies' are likely to dominate.

Changing approaches to service delivery, notably decentralizing services, whether in terms of local offices for services, or on a political basis, with 'neighbourhood town halls' and their very local policy concerns, also have implications for these services. Centralized environmental health offices could encourage specialization within environmental health and give scope for career advancement. In decentralized offices, on the other hand, one staff member might be expected to have expertise in a whole range of environmental health matters. Alternatively, localizing policy making provides a vehicle for a very 'local' public 'say' in environmental health issues, and the creation of 'one stop shops', dealing with all aspects of authority services (as for example in the London Borough of Tower Hamlets) and emphasizing the inter-relationships of service provision.

Opportunities of environmental health departments to investigate environmental factors affecting long-term personal health have led to growing local authority involvement in health promotion. At a wider level, the local authority role in health promotion may now be argued as self-evidently critical, given their ability to facilitate economic and social change in their localities. For some authorities this development may be seen as little more than an extension of their current work, which in no way challenges the policies towards health of other agencies, but rather builds on them, in collaborative fashion. An example of this would be the participation of Welsh Environmental Health departments (22 out of 37 in 1988) in the Welsh Heart Programme, 'Heartbeat Wales'. A national demonstration project, this element involves the presentation of 'Heartbeat awards' to restaurants and canteens, in public and private settings, which meet certain standards and provide particular facilities (Catford and Parrish, 1988).

A more thorough-going approach, which of necessity maintains the collaborative stance, is that taken by those authorities which recognize that their health strategies will be limited without a full picture of the existing state of health within their community, and which link with health authorities to research and report on that state. The report on 'Southwark's Health', produced jointly in 1987 by the London Borough of Southwark's Public Protection Department and the Department of Community Medicine, King's College School of Medicine and Dentistry, 'identifying the roles and clarifying the actions that the council can take in order to improve the health of its population', is a major example of such an exercise (Barnes and Bickler, 1987). Presented as part of the 'development of closer working relationships between the two departments', the report gives major pointers to action. For example, with one in six of the deaths in Southwark resulting from smoking, 'there is more disease and death in Southwark attributable to smoking than any other single avoidable environmental factor' (Barnes and Bickler, p. 47).

Working essentially to draw together and review pre-existing data, the report also draws attention to where basic information on aspects of the community's health is still lacking, or where local authority effectiveness is impeded through lack of powers. For example, 'at least 20% of the population of Southwark is black or from an ethnic minority group, and the 1981 census showed that 17% of the population were born outside the UK' (Barnes and Bickler, p. 41). There is, however, no routinely collected local information on the health of ethnic minorities. In line with national trends, the number of food poisoning cases notified in Southwark was rising, with 'inadequate hygiene awareness and poor controls available to local authorities over the opening of new food businesses . . . central to this' (Barnes and Bickler, p. 52).

For other authorities, widening their health concerns into the health promotion field may provide opportunities to challenge current perceptions of health, and the nature and quality of existing (NHS) provision in a less-than-collaborative, even vociferously critical fashion. Oxford City Council's Health Liaison Officer, speaking on 'local authorities and health' at a conference in 1984, noted cheerfully that

> We do not define health narrowly and we do not mind poking our nose into health authority business,

continuing with the implication that without an element of conflict, neither authority (health authority nor local government) would be doing their job 'in advocating the health of the people in their area' (Fryer, 1987).

Oxford City Council's approach has been assertive, in the sense of emphasizing the importance of its health-orientated work within council committee structures as well as seeking maximum publicity for its health role. Its 'health liaison committee' became merged with its Environmental Control committee, to add a new dimension to the Council's work, and policies have stressed the need for wide contact with its population on health issues, with, for example, health newsletters circulated to every household. Encouragement of recreational programmes has been accompanied by more formal approaches, such as the appointment of designated officers for key health promotion tasks, such as smoking prevention and AIDS liaison. The funding programme is significant in a District Council's budget but not large, Fryer (1987, p. 31) notes spending of £50 000, and an ongoing grants programme to encourage initiatives of £20 000 in 1986–87.

An implicitly critical view of 'mainstream' health services is also expressed by those local authority members advocating not merely that they expand their role in health promotion, but that they pay attention specifically to 'ill health' in their area. Morley (1987), of Sheffield City Council, argues that local authorities 'appear to have placed preventative health care on a secondary policy plateau', and identifies a key local authority role to be re-established, given that 'the NHS appears to have prioritised its available resources heavily in favour of treating the symptoms of ill health rather than preventing its causes'. In arguing in favour of this re-establishment, Morley goes beyond discussion of principle to the practicalities that will face any authority taking this route, and the managerial implications which flow from identifying and maintaining enthusiasm about new priorities.

Once the authority has been able to define and identify the nature and distribution of ill health in its area, the question of what the local authority 'actually wants to achieve' is posed. Morley provides a warning that some authorities' health strategies may read as so all-embracing that they are unlikely to give any clear lead as to priority, and may lead to disappointment and frustration if advance on all or most fronts simultaneously does not occur. Questions needing to be answered and translated into managerial action include:

Does the local authority want to prevent risks to everybody's health or to concentrate on those already with the worst health or groups of those most at risk of preventable ill-health or a mixture of the alternatives?

Does the local authority want to concentrate on certain types of preventable ill health? (Morley, 1987, p. 55)

Morley continues to provide a framework for further policy planning and implementation familiar in the context of local government corporate management styles: the need to formulate clear policy objectives (such as the reduction of deaths from home accidents by 25% by 1995); the need to set operational objectives arising from these for each of the authority's departments; and the importance of identifying a strategy in the sense of identifying the means whereby objectives are translated into action. Further questions posed or implied show the extent to which adopting a health strategy must be interdepartmental in working terms, and involve 'hard choices'; not simply requiring the generation of worthy statements and the agreement of existing departments to 'play their part'. These include whether the authority will need to initiate departmental or committee structural change; whether the authority will operate essentially alone or in collaboration with others; and, probably central, what will be the balance in policy direction and delivery between education and direct intervention.

In examining the issue of which should be the authority's 'lead department' for the strategy, Morley notes in passing that 'in any case it is probable that new employees with specialist skills will be required to complement the existing skills and specialisms already in the Council' (Morley, 1987, p. 58). Arguably, this aspect of the availability – indeed the existence – of a supply of experienced and skilled workers embracing the philosophy of the 'new public health' is more critical than is here presented. Given shortages of professional staffs for other key areas for local government, the 'pool' of such people will not be large, and the expectations of what they will deliver (particularly if they are being seen to challenge hitherto dominant medical models of health and illness) will be high. Some strategies may thus be at risk for a lack of suitable staff or, where they may need to challenge the internal policies of other authority departments, for a lack of suitable staff of sufficiently high status. Some interesting opportunities may exist here for health authority/local authority joint appointments (as with the AIDS Liaison officer post in Oxford, the first in the UK, jointly funded by the DHA and the City Council), or more interestingly, for secondment to local government from health services ranks, even though for some local authority members the latter might be seen to reduce the 'cutting edge' of the policy.

The move into an interest in ill health may be seen as appropriate and inevitable, or, by 'empire building', may simply reflect anxiety not to lose those health responsibilities which authorities still retain. Either way, Morley's message is that local authority health strategies have to be **comprehensive**. To compartmentalize such developments would be to miss the essential point that primary health care questions arise within a range of services, and that responses which are solely departmentally based may be insufficient. Local health strategists have therefore to live with the associated likelihood of overlap of services and recognize the need for sensitivity in co-ordinating intra-authority health related efforts. Even in authorities where health strategies have been formulated to divide up into manageable – and deliverable – programme areas for action, the potential both for overlap and for omission is continuous.

Slough Borough Council's Strategy, recognizes that a 'water-tight', that is, a departmentally-based, approach to health concerns, based on existing departmental structures, will lead to gaps in the provision of health services. It identifies three Programme areas of work, going beyond the 'obvious' committee concerns of environmental health and housing, to include, for example, the authority's personnel committee (Thomson, undated). These are:

1. Area I – the Council's own services and the Council as an employer; involves departmental health target setting, a 'health habit scheme', including healthy eating within the council's catering, employees' fitness testing and an exercise promotion programme; a no smoking policy; and development of a 'comprehensive Occupational Health Service';
2. Area II – Community health promotion and development; involves health protection work, such as pollution control, work on private sector housing repair and fitness, (given impetus by internal reorganization to create a specialist 'domiciliary division'), food hygiene; and health promotion, including encouraging leisure facility use, promoting campaigns concerning alcohol consumption, developing health educational work and promoting occupational health policies among outside employers;
3. Area III – Liaison with other health and health-related bodies servicing the borough; involves the extension of and strengthening of existing contacts with health authorities.

The comprehensiveness of a health strategy is illustrated by these extracts which, standing alone, might nevertheless be seen to demand a particular focus, or theme, as a means of tying in all the disparate but critical policy and service strands. Such a theme does exist for such local authorities, and may itself be seen as a key factor in encouraging local authorities to embark on a high profile approach to health issues. This is the World Health Organization's (WHO) global strategy, 'Health For All by the Year 2000', with its 38 targets set as steps for health for all. In conjunction with this, the WHO's 'Healthy Cities' project, begun in 1986, aims to develop a European network of cities, developing their own strategies, defining local targets and implementing action through various projects. Thus, the above example of an authority's strategy has as its focus 'making Slough a "Healthy City" by the target year 2000'.

Beardshaw (1987), whilst noting that 'the WHO's rhetoric is notoriously difficult to grasp', argues that the aims of this global strategy have provided 'a much broader field for action than most medically determined agenda'; and that whilst some degree of 'bandwagon effect' exists, the current interest in health promotion is 'more than cosmetic'. A Local Authority Health Network now exists which includes the 'UK Healthy Cities Network', an initiative taken in six cities – Oxford, Manchester, Sheffield, Leeds, Coventry and Liverpool – with the intention of adopting and implementing the 38 WHO targets, subject to local conditions.

A key feature of local authority associations with these strategies has been the growth of moves, for example in Sheffield and in Stoke on Trent, to establish local health profiles. These may be defined as statements on the present health of the population together with recommended courses of action to improve health before embarking upon a series of health-based initiatives. In practice these follow the lines discussed above for the London Borough of Southwark. As a rationale for new health initiatives which go beyond the 'medically determined agenda', the research and reporting of these profiles has far-reaching implications. These profiles tend to confirm existing opinions and feelings about geographical patterns of health inequalities, with a consequent focus for discussion on targeting. Even so, the specialized nature of such work may imply a limit as to the number of authorities which can provide or buy in, alone or jointly with others, the necessary statistical and analytical expertise. Circular (88) 64, referred to above, may in practice be seeking to assert the NHS primacy in this area of data gathering and presentation, by asking authorities to review their arrangements for the promotion and maintenance of health.

Nevertheless, the 'Healthy Cities' strategy, with its implicit promotion of an European wide view of 'health for all', provides a valuable reference point for those authorities seeking major shifts in health provision and for those seeking to make contributions on a lesser scale. Fryer (1988) sees the WHO as giving 'a welcome spur to the new public health', in a review of progress being made by Oxford City Council, in its Healthy City strategy, where the uncompromising aim is 'to offset health inequalities in Oxford'. Association with the WHO strategy, and in particular with the establishment of health profiles, and identification thereby of geographical areas of especial need, may further provide some authorities with an improved base from which to argue for more resources from central government. It may also identify the local authorities involved as a form of pressure group, seeking reliable data, with which to support their cause.

That local authority health strategies have in them an element of pressure group behaviour in relation to the NHS – or at least the potential for such – should not be missed. In some authorities this will be implicit: Slough's documentation refers to the need to consider 'consultation documents, strategic plans, operational plans of the (health) authorities and the annual programme of the Family Practitioner Committee' (Thomson, undated, p. 11). The assumption must be that this strategy will be more than simply educational. For those authorities which are also planning authorities, such a role may be more one of sympathetic support or active encouragement for health authority initiatives which are local or community orientated and innovative in nature, rather than one of restriction or criticism. An example cited by Wilce (1988) is the support of Lambeth Borough Council 'with its continued interest as planning authority for the future development of the site', for the establishment of the Lambeth Community Care Centre as an 'inner city community hospital', which she describes as a 'radical experiment in health care'.

In addition, there are also local authority-commissioned 'inquiries' into NHS provision, such as the 'Local Government Public Inquiry into National Health Service Provision in the Northern Region', published in June 1988 by Northern local authorities and the work of externally-appointed experts. In identifying the degree of health-based deprivation in the Region, and the need for improving health services, the report poses a series of challenges for health services members and managers. It may not be surprising that the Regional Health Authority, the 16 district health authorities and the nine family practitioner committees of the region are recorded as neither cooperating nor giving evidence.

This type of approach, certainly intended to raise issues for debate but critical of local health service performance, may increase once the proposals in 'Working for Patients' have taken effect to cease local authority membership of District Health Authorities (DHAs). The poor quality of the relationships between local authorities and DHAs is a growing theme in some of the literature, whether simply as a result of mutual organizational mistrust, or more specifically, mutual ignorance – structural, ideological, professional and procedural. Nocon (1989) identifies this as one of the most striking aspects of organizations' behaviour, impeding the performance of joint planning.

For many authorities, whether or not they have health strategies delineated, there may also be those areas of service where their own provision is frustratingly interlinked with that of the NHS, and where their perceptions of NHS shortfall are strong, leading them to press health authorities to increase their provision. A major example is in the field of children with special educational needs. Welton and Evans (1986) highlight the implicit tension in the 1981 Education Act, whereby local education authorities are required to take responsibility for statements of children's special educational needs, whilst the availability of some provision to meet those needs lies with the DHA, as in the case of speech therapy, for which demand far exceeds supply.

Local education authorities cannot influence directly the resource allocation of a health authority, and although parents may appeal if unsatisfied regarding the provision of needs, 'the LEA cannot force the DHA to provide'. Welton and Evans also point to areas of possible divergence of interest between health and education authorities regarding the integration of children with special needs into mainstream education. Increased integration may place an additional burden on health authorities in the provision of physiotherapy, whereas if special education is concentrated in a special school or unit the physiotherapy service may be provided in a more cost-effective way and with more specialist facilities.

In this area, local authorities face the brunt of parental concern, whilst having to rely on the health authority for a response. In the area of homelessness, where the health needs of homeless people, whilst never high on agendas, have been receiving increased attention recently, the issue is not so much that of pressurizing another organization to perform, as uncertainty as to the means of co-ordinating the services that do exist. In the 1987 report from the Joint Working Party on Single Homelessness in London Health Sub-group, 'Primary Health Care for Homeless Single People in London: A Strategic Approach', it is the health service that is unequivocally identified as having the major role in organizing the provision of mainstream health services to this group (Bayliss and Logan, 1987). Nevertheless, the implications for local authorities needing to borrow capital for the development of 'a whole range of accommodation' to assist the single homeless, and for increased revenue for the prevention of homelessness by local authority-based support services, such as day centres and meals-on-wheels, are also stressed. The need for more resources for a 'concerted effort between health authorities and local borough councils' is seen as setting the context or 'a proper "Inner Cities Health Care programme" ' (Bayliss and Logan, p. 38), with the implication of some sort of equal partnership, with the rejection of the 'tapering' arrangements of joint finance and demand for joint finance for this group on a permanent basis. The report's description of the current situation in relation to the single homeless (Bayliss and Logan, p. 38) might, for some, be taken as applicable to the state of primary health care for other disadvantaged groups:

> . . . a series of partial, short-term, unco-ordinated inner city health care initiatives, which for the most part reflect the outcome of struggles amongst the various lobbies and interest groups within government and the health service.

Whether as service provider, 'new public health advocate' or lobbyist, those local authorities with social services responsibilities have, with District Health Authorities, anxiously awaited the government's White Paper 'Caring for People' (HMSO, 1989).

The White Paper confirmed acceptance of Griffiths' recommendation that local authorities should assume the leading role in assessing, designing and organizing care for eldery and mentally handicapped people, with resources to be transferred from the social security budget to local authorities to help finance their new role. The implications for the required health element in this provision are yet to be spelled out in detail. The Griffiths report itself has emphasized the extension of training which will be required for such a move, with new demands on the management skills and systems in social services departments, and with the need for closer collaboration between people of differing professional backgrounds.

Inter-relationship with the health service not only remains, but in one area is made more intricate by the announcement of the government intention to create a specific grant for the care of mentally ill people, made available to local authorities through health authorities and 'tied to action plans and targets submitted by social services departments' (Sherman, 1989). Thus, health authorities will be the budget holders for mentally ill people. Local authorities will have to satisfy the health authorities that their community care plans are adequate. Such funds are only identified for mental illness, yet arguably the same arrangement would be appropriate for people with mental handicap, on the assumption that the dominant concern has been inappropriate discharge into an unprepared community.

The levels and methods of funding for these developments are critical, yet the White Paper did little to reassure those concerned with the development. The decision to confer leadership on local authorities may be regarded as a vote of confidence in local government, or as a deliberately impossible task with which they will struggle. The resources demand of these new responsibilities may be such as to deflect attention from the preparation of wider health strategies, running across the spectrum of public service provision. Further doubts as to the local authority role have now arisen, with the announcement of the postponement of key elements of the government's community care plans (Timmins, 1990). The reasons appear to be concern over likely cost levels and local authority unpreparedness.

Even allowing for the continuing uncertainties as to the nature and meaning of 'community care' – analysed recently by Higgins (1989) – the focus of debate on the local authority's health-related role has again been narrowed. The more global aims and aspirations, such as reducing health inequalities and 'health for all by the year 2000', seem to be steadily receding.

The motives for local authorities' development of health strategies have been mixed, producing mixed policy objectives and, arguably, mixed results. This is particularly so where the publication of strategy documents leads to minimal change, or where initial enthusiasm is difficult to maintain after early fervour. These developments seem to have occurred partly from a sense of local authorities' exclusion from a policy-making arena which crucially affects their work; from a desire to have at least a quasi-pressure group role; from seeking the expansion of health resources; and from their awareness of the artificiality of drawing up barriers between provision for 'public' and 'individual' health, as well as from a related desire to protect those health services which they still retain. Given the patchiness of the implementation of such strategies, and their inevitably more 'global' nature than services targeted at particular client groups, the degree of their success must be uncertain, although it is possible to see that the very growth of the ideas of the 'new public health' in local authority hands may at least have been a spur towards encouraging the NHS towards reviewing its public health commitments.

2

Developing service strategies: the transition to community care

Su Kingsley and Robin Douglas

The development of community health services represents an area in which some significant changes are taking place in health and social services. The changes themselves reflect a complex interweaving of ideas about the type of care and service that should be available to people, financial pressures, different organizational arrangements and challenges to the established power structures within and between groupings. They are additionally influenced by the development of organized consumer and service user groups which are increasingly articulate about how their needs should best be met. This is extending the notion of consumerism within these services. The management of these processes of change, whilst maintaining acceptable levels of service, is a particularly demanding task. This chapter will identify a number of the key issues affecting these changes and suggest some of the basic elements of a strategic approach.

There is no easily acceptable definition of 'a community service' – much of the difficulty in the development of these services stems from the variety of definitions that are and can be applied. We will return to this problem of defining a community and hence the nature of community services later. Although we are concerned with services for all people, the experience of service developments outlined in this chapter is drawn from the fields of providing services for mentally handicapped and mentally ill people. The provision of integrated, community based services for the largest group of people with related needs – the elderly – is still very much in its infancy. Although lessons from one service sector cannot be simply transferred to another we believe there is much that can prove useful in the development of more effective strategies for other services. We will begin by identifying details of future services which we hope any service strategy would be able to deliver. This will enable us to clarify some of the managerial tasks which will be required in order to deliver such services. From this, in turn, we will discuss how these tasks should improve our understanding of the roles that managers may play as community care strategies are developed.

THE CONTEXT FOR CHANGE

The background to these evolving changes in psychiatric services is the pattern of services rooted in 19th-century institutionalization. Whilst containment was a key feature of earlier approaches our concerns now focus more on the quality of life, the quality, nature and location of care, and on the rights of all citizens to at least a minimum standard of life. The history of serious neglect of institutional services which provided fodder for the major critiques and enquiries of the 1960s is well known. Enabling legislation (the 1959 Mental Health Act) and subsequent Government policy papers (DHSS 1971, 1975) set directions and suggested some limited aspirations for the development of alternative patterns of care.

We now have a rich and complex infrastructure of services provided by local authority social services, voluntary agencies and the private sector, as well as through the health care system. This provides opportunities for developing community care strategies as alternatives to institutional care, but also poses major problems of integrating the work of different organizations, and creating partnership and collaboration towards agreed ends. The degree and nature of such collaborative endeavour has been subject to much debate, which remains unresolved at the time of writing (Griffiths, 1988). However given existing variations it seems unlikely that a uniform pattern of inter-agency arrangements will result.

The NHS in particular lacked the capacity to plan services before the 1974 re-organization (Levitt, 1976); the complex planning structure that was then introduced focused more on the co-ordination and integration of incremental changes than on the major issues of planning and implementing service shifts. The requirement for consensus and agreement at many levels of NHS organization tended to have the effect of levelling out proposals for major change, leaving only minor readjustments as acceptable to all interests involved. Management in the NHS reflected these patterns. Over the last five years, however, NHS management has moved from consensus administration to general management control. In our view, creating community care services will require a further shift towards the management of organizational processes rather than simply the control of systems and procedures.

THE DEVELOPMENT OF A MANAGEMENT CULTURE

The structure of the NHS shifted in 1982 to focus on units of management. This was greatly strengthened by the introduction of general management two years later, and these initiatives have radically changed the planning capacity of the NHS. They have enabled the creation in most districts of units where the responsibility for an overall pattern of service to a client group is focused (although some districts have retained a split across client groups according to the type of care being received, for example acute/ long-term) and responsibilities for action are consequently much clearer.

The unit manager is in a pivotal position in respect of such changes. It is at unit level that demands for service and demands for change are balanced against the constraints imposed though the District and Region by national priorities and resources. This creates great opportunities for managers and their staff in the unit to develop services, create alliances with other agencies and interest groups, communicate directly with users and potential users of services and advocate resources and recognition of the needs of their client group. It also places managers in an exposed and vulnerable position, where they are likely to experience pressures and demands from all directions. A major challenge of unit management is to achieve a balance between these pressures and demands, and to use their energy to move the service in new directions which will lead to better experiences for the service users.

Similar patterns of development can also be identified in organizations allied to the NHS which will need to be engaged in the process of managing these shifts in service arrangements. Although clearly operating within a wide range of different political environments, a management culture is developing within many local authority social services departments. Concern with more realistic service planning has grown from the initial uncontrolled growth that followed the establishment of Departments as a result of the Seebohm Report (Ministry of Health, 1968) and the decade of resource limitations which superseded growth in the 80s. Voluntary organizations, particularly those organized on a national basis, are also becoming more conscious of a need to manage the costs and quality of their activities – a prerequisite for a more integrated service strategy.

Our introduction has indicated the complex strands and interests which currently form the backdrop to demands for and expectations of change in the priority services. A history of neglect punctuated by the spotlight of scandal has not promoted a climate in which reform is fostered or learning valued. Further there is dissent about appropriate directions for future services, which are more marked in some areas (services for people with mental illness for example) than in others. At the same time pressure for change is increasing, and it is managers at District and Unit level who will be expected to promote the development of new service patterns for priority groups, which focus on strengthening the delivery of care outside large institutions and acute hospital units.

DEVELOPING AN EFFECTIVE RESPONSE

There has been very limited appreciation of the nature of the problem posed by our aspirations to·better community services (Glennerster *et al.*, 1983). It is most frequently described in deceptively simple terms which disguise its true nature as a 'wicked problem' (Rittel and Weber, 1974); moreover, a wicked problem existing in a highly volatile environment. 'Wicked' problems are those to which there is no technical solution, however hard it may be sought, or however much information is brought to bear on the problem. The 'solution' involves making moral and political choices: situations which bureaucratic organizations are poorly prepared for. The development of responses to wicked problems means that organizations need to learn about and reflect on the processes by which such choices can be made, instead of seeking a technical answer which will avoid the issue of choice.

Thus developing community services is not a task which has a simple solution, already tried and tested, which merely needs to be applied to a local context. It is not a bounded problem of making a specific change, reflecting on its impact, and then moving on. Rather it requires the ability to develop the capacity to generate new solutions and, through trying them, learning more about the development process and the organization which could best deliver effective community services.

In this sense dealing with wicked problems is about creating and maintaining real change within the organization which enhances its capacity to learn from experience. In John O'Brien's words approaching wicked problems, developing creative community services, requires us to take cognizance of the three teachers 'ignorance, error and fallibility' (O'Brien, 1987). Thus how managers behave, and the processes by which organizations operate, becomes a much more fundamental question than whether the appropriate structures are in place. Indeed insuring appropriate processes, developing creative working practices and designing enabling structural arrangements that clarify organizational vision, identify the goals and objectives and financial frameworks are the key tasks for management. The problem is not to establish a clearly laid-out strategy like a 'yellow brick road' but rather to provide the means to redefine direction and pace in the light of changing circumstances – an **emergent** rather than **prescribed** approach.

Figure 2.1 shows how managers need to change their focus and

Role		Manager	
	Features of the Environment	Known	Unknown
Subordinate	Known	1. Explicit goal setting	3. Task process and management monitoring
	Unknown	2. Subordinate development	4. Task/group inter and intra personal process management

Figure 2.1 Possible management responses to environmental certainty and uncertainty

behaviour in response to differing levels of certainty and uncertainty within the environment. Goal setting and monitoring (1), together with some developmental activity in relation to staff (2), are often the limits of managerial behaviour. Yet it can be seen from the figure that these activities may be entirely inappropriate in situations characterized by high uncertainty. These require a new approach based on the management of process, concerned with both how the tasks are to be carried out and how people can work together to achieve this, if new developments are to be created and supported.

Organizing to respond to the community

We mentioned earlier the difficulty in developing an unambiguous definition of 'the community'. Volumes of literature describe the community in terms of:

1. communities of interest, need, or shared concerns;
2. geographical locations or neighbourhoods with definable boundaries or associating characteristics;
3. convenient political systems interwoven with needs;
4. a political or value laden construct that implies a range of ideas, such as a reduction in dependence on institutions or professionals; greater control by users over service design, development and management; emphasis on devolution of resources and authority to small localized service units; services run with rather than provided for users, etc.; or
5. a mythical notion of self sufficiency for all but acute and tertiary care (Abrams, 1977).

This wide range of definitions, assumptions and implied values is clearly present in the plans and actions of the organizations and actors involved in the transition processes between institutional and community care, and those trying to inject new vigour into the 'old' community health services. No universally acceptable definition is possible but a recognition of these differences is the prerequisite of a move towards coherency in strategic planning. The manager can enable or facilitate the process of exploring these different definitions. This can be a particularly important task to do on an inter-agency basis where services are jointly planned or managed.

The management issues

A key problem in the development of community services is the scope and variety of needs that the concept of community services includes. This requires us to consider very different groups of people with very diverse needs. Some groups are much more easy to identify and more visible than others; some are more articulate and demanding. Small shifts in need, or the perception of need, may have a major impact on available resources (an example is the rapidly rising 'board and lodgings' payments to elderly people in residential care). The extent of this variation means that it is unlikely that community services can be effectively planned on a unitary basis; disaggregation is necessary in order to break down the many tasks into manageable and discrete elements. What criteria should be used to bring about such a breakdown? Many units have adopted a **client group** division: this is helpful in providing focus, but major questions remain for groups with diverse needs such as elderly people and people with mental illness. Other districts have adopted a **locality** approach, planning all community services on the basis of small, defined population sub-sets. This can be an advantage where other agencies, and especially social services, have also adopted 'patch' based approaches to organizing the delivery of local services. It provides a distinct target group for service development, with allocated resources that may be controlled at local level, and so does much to focus the planning and implementation process. The disadvantage of a locality based approach is the dilution of specialist services and expertise that it entails, which must somehow be built into a wider overall framework. A third, and declining way of organizing responses to the community is on the basis of **services**, for example many social services departments are still organized into residential, day care, domiciliary and fieldwork service groups who plan and deliver care on a relatively independent basis. Clearly this form of separation has many disadvantages and much potential for confusion.

Obtaining useful definitions of need

Commonly the definition of need, particularly in specialized, institutional or acute services, is defined by the service providers. This definition is often couched in terms of a professional diagnosis ('this leg needs mending' or 'that organ needs replacing'). This is often statistically extended to describe a group or population – 'We are likely to have to respond to 100 problems like this in this district per week' – and hence to determine the nature of the service provided. National, local or other normative data are also used to complement this process of service design.

Community based services require a rather more complex model of needs that encompasses the service users' perspectives, hopes and aspirations as well as those of the professionals and managers. Jonathan Bradshaw (1972) suggests a useful notion of normative, comparative, felt and expressed needs, to provide a framework for the debate about service design and priorities.

However, having an agreed language for the description of need is only a part of the picture. Developing community services by relying on a definition of local needs could be a recipe for disaster, encouraging an expectation that unmet needs may now be responded to by community services. This could lead to considerably increased pressure on existing services and subsequently more dissatisfied people who are involved in giving or receiving service. The underlying assumption here is that community services cannot be managed within a 'demand led' model but must be rationed, that is planned, organized and operated from the 'supply' side. The nature and availability of resources thus becomes the prime determinant of service design.

We would suggest that while neither needs nor supply alone should direct the strategy for developing community care, both have their place. The unit manager's job is to ensure that there is clarity in the planning process in respect of the contribution of needs assessment and service review. Those asked or required to contribute to the planning and management of these services must be clear what authority they have for decisions and priorities and what is retained by managers. The consultation process is a mine field in which many community care strategies have ground to a halt through lack of clarity in this area.

Co-ordinating diverse organizational and individual goals

It is likely that the diversity of objectives pursued by individuals and organizations involved in community health and community care strategies has been one of the most significant negative influences on their successful implementation. Much energy and effort appears to go into attempting to negotiate agreements about overall organizational goals as a precursor to service development. This effort is highly likely to be unsuccessful. The existence of a number of different participating organizations requires us to suppose that they have differences in their aims, sometimes only in degree but usually enough to ensure that at some stage in planning disagreements will occur. This recogition can be helpful in reducing the effort to achieve total organizational agreements, replacing this with 'good enough' agreements to allow service planning and activities to go ahead. An important stage in this process of at least understanding these differences is to separate ends and means – outcome goals or objectives, and service goals or methods of care. Agreement that is often possible about ends is often confused with discussions about means or vice versa; NHS staff implicitly or explicitly accused by social workers of promoting a 'medical model' of services is an example of this process. Here the discussion about means ('We don't like the way you organize that hostel') is used to obscure a real dispute, that may or may not exist in reality, about goals ('We disagree about what we think you are trying to achieve for these handicapped people).

The manager's task must be to ensure that discussions, reports or papers do not waste effort in attempting an impossible integration of organizational goals and do not allow emotional debates to obscure potential areas of agreement.

STRATEGIES FOR CHANGE

Basic values

Many changes in health care have been heavily influenced by developments in professional expertise, shifts in interests and advances in medical technology. Whilst expertise and technology have contributed to demands for change in priority group care, the greater impetus is now a social one, concerning changing public and professional opinions about the appropriate way to provide care for dependent adults. One starting point in a strategy for change is to consider the **outcome** which is being aimed for (Elmore, 1982): in this case, changes which lead to improvements in the experiences of service users. There may be, of course, a number of alternative end states, each of which is illustrated in current services in different places. Some alternative goals include 'cheaper services', 'transfer of care to the family (effectively women carers)', and 'a wider choice of services'. Our analysis is grounded in an assumption that the final arbiter of the effectiveness of a service should be the person who uses it, and consequently our test of its effectiveness must rest on the impact a service has on the user's life and his/her experiences.

In order to achieve significant shifts in service users' experiences it has been argued that change must be both **principled** and **systematic** (Towell and Kingsley, 1988). Any strategy for service development will need to ensure that attention is paid to both these aspects.

What principles might be used to inform community care strategies? How can or should they be developed? Within the area of social care for priority groups the issue of values and principles is much more confused than for medical care for acutely ill individuals, where although some of the means may be disputed, there is much more general acceptance of the ends or outcomes of treatment. The 'priority' groups have been identified precisely because they include groups of people who are not highly valued within most industrial societies: elderly, mentally and physically disabled people and people with mental illnesses who are commonly considered to be unproductive and dependent.

Two clear strands have emerged from the experience of Districts which have tried to develop a shared value base for their service development process. First there is much benefit in paying attention to the creation of such a local value base (Kingsley and Towell, 1988). Activities focused on articulating local aspirations can serve as a means to engage diverse local interests and help in identifying common ground. Gaining commitment to a core of commonly held aspirations can create a powerful force for change. A second important strand in developing principled change for priority group clients is the work on normalization, developed in North America during the last decade. This has been powerfully expressed in the UK through the work on 'An Ordinary Life' for people with mental handicaps; and the publications and training workshops of the Campaign for Mentally Handicapped People (CMH) and CMHERA (Tyne and O'Brien, 1981).

The values underpinning normalization are now being applied to services for other client groups, and are particularly appropriate when considering services for elderly people (Kings Fund, 1987).

A vision of future services

So far we have dealt with some of the ideas and issues clustered around the notion of change as 'principled'. Aspirations for change provide the outlines on which a vision of the future can be drawn. The challenge for service managers and providers is to create a process for linking the known present and the hoped for future. This will mean identifying an initial direction and action plan, ensuring that progress is initiated and maintained, and monitoring the outcomes regularly. The route will not be straightforward: it will require careful interpretation of signposts along the way, and a creative approach to obstacles and diversions, which may require alterations in the route without deviating from the ultimate goal. Some will argue that the 'vision of service' is not the terrritory for the manager, that this is the province of the professional or carer and the task of management is to enable them to determine the process and outcome goals (means and ends) and then provide the resources and operational support to ensure that goals may be achieved. Our belief is that managers not only have a right to be involved in determining the nature of the services, they have a clear responsibility to develop their vision, explore their assumptions about the 'principles' of the service and make explicit the values that they wish to be promoted by any service for which they are to be held ultimately accountable. The development of strategy represents a multi-dimensional map of the territory between present and future; a map which we know is incomplete in many aspects, but which represents an interweaving of several different elements of change.

The elements of a community care strategy

It is possible to conceptualize the development of service strategies by the interactions between a series of principal areas of concern (Figure 2.2). Each influences the other and is influenced by features of the local, organizational and wider context in which it is sited.

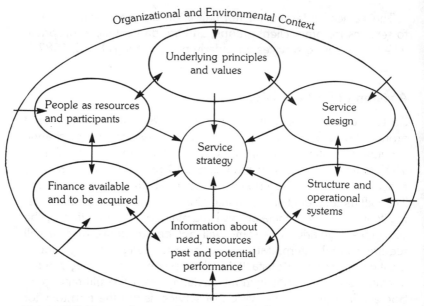

Figure 2.2 Principal areas of concern in developing service strategies

Together they enable the service strategy itself to surface. Clearly a manager cannot do all of this. His/her role is to ensure that all these concerns are rigorously addressed and to manage the processes that lead to 'good enough' agreements to move the strategy ahead. The **processes** of working on these six main areas will in themselves contribute either negatively or positively to the progress of the strategy – 'the medium is the message' – there is no starting tape. Therefore, the skill in managing in these uncertain areas must lie in the ability to maintain a clear **personal** framework of goals, values and priorities, whilst being **open** to influence from individuals and groups within and outside the participating organizations. If ideas of openness, trust and recognition of individuality are basic principles of the service system, should they not also be part of the management processes? Is it possible to deliver a 'principled' service through organizations operating according to a different value base?

The service strategy will be composed of a number of sub-strategies, each focused on ensuring the co-ordination and integration of the major areas of concern: values and principles, service design, people, finance, systems and information.

In this respect developing an effective community care strategy requires managers to extend the nature of general management into the realms of 'process' management: managing by enabling rather than by objectives.

SOME PROBLEMS IN EXECUTION

Whilst we are now able to define these essential components for creating real changes in services, experience suggests that this has rarely been achieved in practice. There are examples of Districts where significant progress is being made, and these examples bear out our contention that change is required simultaneously on a number of strategic fronts. However, so far such Districts are the exception rather than the rule, as recent reports from the House of Commons Select Committee on Social Services (HMSO 1985) and the Audit Commission (1986) have pointed out. Both these reports express disappointment with the lack of progress towards community based services and the barriers to improving levels of service to priority care groups in the community (i.e. elderly people, people with mental handicaps, people suffering mental illness and younger people with physical disabilities). Both reports point out the 'patchy' nature of developments that have taken place. In other words, they highlight areas of good practice which have not so far been generalized.

Misunderstanding the problem

While the Select Committee drew attention particularly to the problems it perceived as deriving from insufficient financial resources, and a lack of 'vision' for the future – a point made more forcibly by Stuart Etherington and Nick Bosanquet (1985) – the Audit Commission's primary concern is with the fragmented organizational structure of current services, which makes collaboration difficult and creates disincentives to community care in some cases. Lack of resources and investment in change, complex and conflicting structures and lack of direction are all clearly major difficulties to be overcome in achieving change. However, they are also symptoms of a more fundamental issue which must be appreciated if change is to be more than marginal and ultimately to be made to 'stick'. We have referred earlier to the concept of developing community care services as a 'wicked problem', that is, a problem which is connected to values and is therefore essentially moral rather than technical in nature. Many of our difficulties derive from a failure to distinguish effectively between moral and technical problems and therefore to try to apply technical solutions to problems of value and choice. If the development of community care is properly understood as a moral problem, it becomes clear that the managerial task is not to identify the correct technical resources for its resolution but rather to create a collaborative process for all the 'stakeholders' to contribute to the choices which will have to be made. This must operate within an acceptable set of 'ground rules' that encourages contributions and does not raise unrealistic expectations in terms of degree of consultation or resource availability.

Who holds the strings?

Community based services are not simply a shift of service to a different site. The development of community services implies a real change in the nature of the service itself. As the Audit Commission's report summed it up, this change is essentially one from a **caring** to an **enabling** service. This will mean a significant shift in the balance of power from the organization delivering the service (providing care) to the user who is increasingly conceptualized as a consumer, with rights, abilities and opportunities to make choices about how, when and where services should be available to them to support their daily lives. Power shifts are not easy to negotiate, neither are they painless. However if we are to take seriously the key accomplishment of respect for service users as individuals it is a crucial shift to achieve. An intermediate example is provided by the Kent Community Care scheme where field social workers have responsibility for a local budget, which they can use to buy in services which maintain elderly people in their own homes. Crossroads Care Attendant schemes are based on the premise that the care providers do what the client requires of them, whatever that may be; and no more, no less. Experiments in user control of a social club budget have proved successful and empowering in N. Derbyshire, and could well be repeated elsewhere.

Different planning for different services

Throughout this chapter we have stressed that the key task required of managers in transition to community care is to ensure that processes are in place which enable the organization to learn and adapt itself to new situations; and we have pointed out that this requires that managers' first concerns should be to create an environment in which their staff are enabled to develop new ideas and try out new ways of doing things. The outcomes of these activities – the processes of involvement, planning, experiment and learning – will always need to be tailored to the specific situation in which they are developing. The planning of mental health services in Area A will probably look quite different from the process adopted in Area B, although B may have learned from looking at A's experiences. Similarly in B, planning for mental handicap services and services for elderly people will each differ significantly from the process worked out for the mental health service. There are no blue-prints for this sort of development: learning is a key aspect, but the learning must focus on such questions as 'What is it that we might learn from X?', 'How might we utilize this learning?' and 'How can we learn from other services?' rather than attempting direct transfers of the outcome of a development process from one area or service to another.

The management role – a checklist of action

As a means of summarizing the points made within this chapter, Table 2.1 lists areas that may be of concern for managers in developing their personal strategies to enable an effective organizational approach to developing community health services or community care.

Although no single unit strategy is likely to match that of another, the overall 'agenda' to which they work should be very similar: it is highly probable that the same issues will need to be addressed at some time, but it is the order and intensity of such activity that will differ. The skilful manager will have a map of the terrain, much of which is likely to be known to their management team, and the ability to monitor progress and maintain organization and individual momentum.

Table 2.1 Examples of management and managers' tasks in responding to strategic issues

Strategic Issue	Implication for Unit	Focus for Management Action
1) Agreeing organizational and individual goals	What degree of agreement is possible/necessary? Need to enable inter-organizational clarification of ends and means. Integrating NHS, LA, FPC, VOLORGS and other organizational goals.	Identify agreement and dispute points. Identify own terms and objectives. Encourage 'principle' discussion. Obtain 'good enough' agreements. Developing public statements/missions. Negotiation/conciliation.
2) Clarifying needs and resources	Determining sources and criteria for identifying needs. Assessing effectiveness of services. Identifying values and principles underlying the application of need criteria.	Ensure existence of active data systems. Negotiate contribution from different organizations and individuals. Monitor existing services for use, acceptability, levels of performance. Creating capacity of learning from experience.
3) Structuring organizations for community care	Clarifying notions of 'community'. Integrating different organizational approaches. Delegating authority, responsibility and resources.	Identify ranges and definitions of community and CC used in own and others' organizations. Communicating with other organizations on their organizational arrangements and plans. Develop criteria to judge appropriateness of organizational design.

4) Funding the services	Maintaining old facilities/services. Developing new facilities/services. Acquiring new/additional funding.	Identify creative financial strategies. Establish means to cost/evaluate community based service modes (e.g. balance of care model).
5) Developing organizational learning	Ensuring organizations involved learn from their experiences. Enabling individuals to contribute to the learning process in terms of the quality of service delivery and effectiveness of the strategic processes. 'Learning to learn.'	Provide reflection/review mechanisms to learn from the strategies in action. Identify staff and other people who can usefully contribute to the strategies.
6) Interlinking strategies	Need for coherence in strategic activities, time planning and resource access for the strategic process. Reviewing impacts of additional workload.	Develop personal priorities and time budget for strategy. Provide subordinates with sufficient time/space/encouragement to contribute to strategies and maintain existing services.

John Stewart (1986) helpfully describes three elements of effective strategic management:

1. *Strategic thinking* The capacity to see general patterns in the complexity of the daily activity, choose significant actions and events from many distractions, work out policies and activities that will have maximum input and identify the opportunities for change.
2. *Strategic leadership* The ability to give direction and momentum towards the organizational goals, including an assessment of the impacts of new policies, the impact of change on the organization and creating effective responses to unexpected developments.
3. *Strategic organizational development* The process of enabling the organization to learn from the experiences of change and positioning itself to increase its overall learning capacity in the light of a continually changing environment. This area is considered much more an 'art' than a science.

General managers must utilize fully these three elements, with a focus on the content issues that we have identified throughout this chapter, if they are to establish strategies for community health services and community care. This is an extremely difficult task, but one with enormous implications for improved services, more efficient use of resources and more satisfied customers.

3

Patterns of management in community units

Gillian Dalley

Community health services have a chequered history; many would argue that it has been one of marginality and associated low status, pointing to the fact that they have been variously moved from one agency to another and have been overshadowed by other, more prestigious sectors of the health and social services establishments. At the inception of the National Health Service, it was decided that they should continue under local authority control, as they had been in the past. After the health service reorganization in 1974 they became the responsibility of the newly established Area Health Authorities. It is only in recent years, however, that they have developed a clear identity of their own within the formal structure of the NHS.

ORGANIZATIONAL CHANGE AFTER 1974

The National Health Service Act 1973 marked a profound change in the structure and organization of the health service. The Act integrated hospitals and community health services into one administrative unit. In 1974 the 625 different bodies (DHSS/PSSC 1978) which had run the NHS up to that point (mostly hospital management committees) were abolished and administration was organized on a geographically defined basis in terms of Regions, Areas and Districts, coinciding as far as possible with local authority boundaries. At the same time, local authorities passed over responsibility to the new health authorities for certain community health services (such as health visiting and district nursing) while local authorities became responsible for the provision of social work services within hospitals, clinics and general practice. Management of the health services within the new authorities was based on a system which came to be known as 'consensus management'; the heads of four strands of functional leadership or line management (medicine, nursing, finance and administration) came together as a management team, with no one individual having overall authority but with the team being responsible for decision making and accountable to the tier above it.

The 1974 reorganization, it has been argued (Klein, 1983), was seen by policy-makers as an opportunity to introduce modern, rational planning into the service. Alaszewski, Tether and Robinson (1982) saw the key themes as being centralization and managerial efficiency. Centralized monitoring and guidance was intended to ensure a more even distribution of resources along with health authorities' compliance with central government's priorities. Nevertheless, there were difficulties. As Barbara Castle, then Secretary of State at the DHSS, said in 1976:

> One of the biggest challenges to effective democratic government is how to reconcile two potentially conflicting aims: central government must be able to establish and promote certain essential national priorities, while the local agencies of government should have the maximum scope for making their own local choices in the light of their local needs. (DHSS, 1976)

Before the end of the decade, those difficulties were being increasingly recognized. A Royal Commission was established to look into the workings of the NHS; it reported in 1979 and drew attention to unresolved problems of organization and policy implementation (DHSS, 1979a).

In 1979, the new Conservative government published the policy document, 'Patients First' (DHSS, 1979b) which claimed to represent a move away from targets, norms and centralization. It stressed the need for local assessment of need and argued for the delegation of decision-making power because

> the closer decisions are taken to the local community and to those who work directly with patients, the more likely it is that patients' needs will be their prime objective. (DHSS, 1979b)

These views were later confirmed in the circular HC (80)8 which provided guidance for another round of reorganization. This heralded the abolition of Area Health Authorities, the establishment of smaller, District Health Authorities (DHAs) and the formation of units of management within districts. In the interests of speedy and effective decision making, there was to be no tier between the units as envisaged and the District Health Authority. The structure was to be clear, simplified and, wherever possible, was to correspond with 'natural' socio-geographical contours and local authorities (although it was Area Health Authorities which had been most often conterminous with local authorities).

From the point of view of the community health services the circular was particularly significant. As well as requiring the establishment of units of management for the first time, it also laid out a range of examples of how they might be constituted. It suggested that they could be any of the following: institutional (based on a single large hospital, or group of smaller hospitals); community based (community health services); client-group based (all the services for a particular client group gathered together in one unit); or geographical (to include small institutions and community health services within a defined geographical area). Until this point the community health services had not had a very distinct identity. They had been shunted between agencies. Under local authority control they had been somewhat overshadowed by the other services for which the local authorities were responsible (housing, child welfare and so on); on coming under health authority control, they had tended to be dominated by their – arguably – more powerful and prestigious partners, the acute hospital services. Now for the first time, the opportunity was being offered for them to be organized and managed discretely.

The changes proposed in the circular came into effect in 1982. Area Health Authorities were abolished and the new units of management within districts came into being. A glance at the 'Hospital Year Book' for 1984 [IHSM, 1984] shows that most districts had decided to establish units dealing wholly or predominantly with the community health services.

Within the units, the system of consensus management was maintaned, with nursing, medicine, administration and finance being led or managed separately, but in parallel. This, however, was not to last. In 1983, Roy Griffiths presented the results of his inquiry into the management of the NHS (DHSS, 1983). His chief recommendation was the introduction of general management throughout the system. This meant that consensus management would be replaced by the appointment of a single 'general manager' or 'chief executive' at each structural level who would have sole responsibility for what went on below him or her. Thus regions, districts and units would all have general managers heading the service at each level. Central government accepted the Griffiths recommendations and in 1984 general managers began to be appointed, phased in gradually from the top. Unit General Managers (UGMs) began to come into post during 1985.

GENERAL MANAGEMENT IN COMMUNITY UNITS

UGMs came into post charged with a duty to establish clear structures of management and accountability within their units. A survey conducted in the late autumn of 1986 of all English health authorities showed that most community units were adopting strikingly similar approaches to their internal organization (King's Fund Centre, 1987b). Fundamentally these seemed to indicate that the general manager has ultimate power of decision making in all that goes on below him or her and is fully accountable to the general manager immediately above for those decisions. Equally important to the principles of general management is the concept of the general manager, that is, the manager is appointed irrespective of professional background to manage a range of services and staff of differing professions. The appointment is made on the basis of evident skills in management and leadership. Another crucial component in a generally managed organization is the process of objective-setting and the monitoring of progress towards those objectives. The organization should have 'a sense of mission', know where it is going and be able to monitor performance towards those ends.

How then did the new community unit general managers plan to incorporate the essential principles of general management into the new structures and strategies that they intended to introduce? According to the King's Fund survey (1987b), many of them planned to introduce some form of decentralization. Of 166 health authorities replying to a questionnaire circulated to all English health authorities, over two-thirds (140) suggested that they were likely to do so or had already done so.

Decentralizing the community health services can be seen to be appropriate for two separate but interconnected reasons. First, one of the chief characteristics of the services is that they are dispersed in a spatial, geographical sense. It can be convincingly argued that dispersed services of this sort are likely to be more amenable to effective management and organization at the local level than if directed from a central headquarters bureaucracy as had often happened in the past. Second, one element in general management, as has been noted, is concerned with delegating decision making downwards; it builds on the philosophy expressed in 'Patients First' that decisions are best taken as close to patients and their local communities as possible. Thus it would be possible to combine the organization of the services on a decentralized basis – from local offices based in health centres and clinics throughout the geographical area of the District Health Authority – with a structure of delegated or devolved general management within the unit (that is, at sub-unit level) that matched this physical decentralization.

From responses to the questionnaire it seems that this approach has been widely adopted; 140 authorities replied that they were planning to decentralize the organization of their services in the physical sense. Of a range of five possible options suggested in the questionnaire, a third said that decentralization was to involve management, service delivery, budgets, planning and information. More than half mentioned at least four of these options. Over 100 districts also planned to appoint 'locality managers' to be responsible for services in local areas. Of these districts, more than half intended to carry the general management principle down through the unit too, so that locality managers would also be general managers of their localities, not simply line managers of one professional group or another.

THE AIMS AND OBJECTIVES OF DECENTRALIZED COMMUNITY UNITS

On the basis of statements of objectives and strategies received from a number of health authorities (for example, Islington, Croydon, Wandsworth, South Sefton, North Staffordshire) and from the participation of more than 40 health authorities in a conference looking at the decentralization of community health services, it is possible to talk with some authority about the aims and objectives of those community units committed to a policy of decentralization (King's Fund Centre, 1987c).

Islington DHA's Community and Continuing Care Unit, for example, outlined eight essential elements in its objectives:

1. The need to provide a flexible and accessible service to meet local needs and to take account of environmental and social factors;
2. To work as closely as possible with services provided elsewhere in the health authority;
3. To optimize interagency co-ordination and co-operation between health and other statutory and voluntary organizations;
4. To recognize that community health services should make it easy for patients and clients to be provided with appropriate care in their local environment;
5. To provide services which could enhance primary healthcare team working and avoid duplication and confusion;
6. To recognize that the consumer, as patient or client, has a right to comment on the local health service and the quality of services delivered;
7. To provide management arrangements which encourage community staff to work as a team, and to remove administrative obstacles which inhibit staff from delivering care in the best possible way;
8. To enable resources and decision making to be devolved to the point of service delivery, to set targets for staff and to enable managers to let staff know how well they are doing. (Dalley and Shephard, 1987)

This was the list of objectives spelt out by a unit general manager who was about to embark on the decentralization of his unit. They represented a first attempt to apply the principles of new-style general management to a unit structure which itself had only been in existence for a few years.

The declared principles that seem to have emerged across the country over the last three or so years seem to be those of accountability, responsiveness, co-ordination and co-operation, participation and appropriateness. Thus the system of general management, and the requirements that that imposes in terms of objectives, accountability and consumer satisfaction (the other major emphasis in Griffiths), seems to have combined with a commitment to principles related to definitions of 'quality' in service provision (Maxwell, 1984). Thus community units are concerned to provide services which adjust in response to changing needs. In furtherance of this, they seek to involve consumers in the planning and reviewing of services. In addition, they give explicit recognition to the problems that have beset community services over the years – namely, the problems of interagency and interprofessional co-operation – and seek to overcome them.

There is an explicit assumption that by organizing and managing services locally, the principles outlined above can be more easily achieved. Stress is placed on the importance of gathering information at local level, and then analysing it and responding to it locally. Information is defined broadly. It may include socio-demographic information deriving from census data; morbidity and mortality data; rates of service uptake; the deployment of local authority and health authority staff and facilities – but it also includes the 'soft' and informal knowledge that local workers and residents have about the locality. A highly textured profile of local areas can be built up from the pooling of all forms of information, with the intention of matching resources to the needs thus revealed. As particular or special needs are demonstrated in one locality, the unit should be able to deploy staff and other resources accordingly. Decisions about shifting resources in this way can be made explicitly and equitably, on the basis of sound information. In relation to the problems of fragmentation and lack of co-operation and co ordination, the assumption is that by encouraging front-line staff working for the variety of agencies at local level to build relationships and resolve problems themselves, without resort to their centralized management hierarchies, difficulties will be overcome.

While the aims of decentralization may be clear, the assumptions upon which they are based (that an approach based on 'localness' is a more efficacious means of achieving the objectives than any other) are to a large extent untested. Of course, the concepts of 'community' and 'neighbourhood' have been widely adopted in recent years in social work and in political thinking (NISW 1982; Hambleton and Hoggett, 1984) and have undoubtedly influenced thinking in other fields, but, again, they are concepts which are largely unproven. Nevertheless, in the case of the health service, given the twin facts of general management and the geographical spread of the community services, there is an appealing logic in proposing a structure and system based on principles of decentralization.

THE IMPLEMENTATION OF LOCALITY MANAGEMENT

Obviously the test of the locality approach is in its implementation. In relation to this, it is important to remember the context in which such implementation takes place. The health service has been subject to considerable change over recent years; the task of introducing 'yet another' change may be complicated by resistance or lack of enthusiasm of the staff involved – or it may be difficult to get a new system to take root in a wider organization which is still trying to find its identity. Further, one of the chief characteristics of the community health services is that they are located in an 'uncontrolled' environment; they coexist with many other services and their clients are subject to the influences of many other services. The health service does not have control over outcomes in the community in the same way that it does, in theory, within an nclosed hospital environment. The effectiveness, say, of changes in the health visiting service might be confounded by deleterious changes in the local authority's housing policy or central government's social security policy.

That having been acknowledged, many community units have proceeded with their plans for implementation. Locality profiles have been drawn up and localities (or areas, or sectors, or neighbourhoods – the terminology varies) have been defined. Managers have been appointed to head the new localities and staff have been deployed within the localities, based as far as possible on information deriving from the locality profiles but subject to continuous monitoring and review as the process of information collection and analysis becomes more sophisticated. First steps have been taken in establishing a public identity for localities – in some cases (for example, North Staffordshire and Exeter) with the establishment of locality forums – and in forming links with other local services and agencies, such as social service departments and GPs.

Nevertheless, various issues have been thrown up during the course of implementation; many of these have been discussed in some detail (Dalley, 1989a). A number of them relate to the introduction and management of change – problems which would be likely to occur whatever system was being introduced. Others, however, have been related to the specific characteristics of decentralization and locality management. Before examining some of both kinds of issues, it is perhaps useful to list some of the more detailed objectives of locality management. They can be listed as follows:

1. multi-disciplinary approach which is client-focused
2. there should be locally based
   (a) decision making and management
   (b) identification of needs
   (c) planning
   (d) service organization and delivery
3. collaborative
   (a) across agency boundaries
   (b) across units
   (c) across professions
4. consumerist
   (a) listening to and valuing consumer views
   (b) involving consumers in planning
5. high quality services
   (a) appropriate
   (b) responsive
   (c) efficient/effective
   (d) equitable

Progress towards some of these objectives is more readily achieved than towards others. It is relatively easy to achieve objectives that are based on formal policy decisions. Many units have secured the support of their health authorities in terms of formal decisions about decentralization and have gone ahead and introduced the relevant structures and managerial appointments. Thus in terms of the objectives listed above, there has been significant progress towards introducing locally based decision making and management, planning and service organization and delivery. Some of the other objectives – those of building cooperative relationships with other agencies and professionals, and of building in a consumerist perspective – remain goals to work towards, along with the goal of high quality services.

But even where progress has been made, a number of important issues have emerged. First, are all the issues related to the introduction and management of change. Significant structural reorganization has been met with varying degrees of acceptance or resistance by staff according to the level of the organization at which they are located, or according to the expectations they have vested in the change (Dalley, 1989a). Those whose own personal position seems to be threatened (for example, middle managers) tend to be hostile; front-line practitioners are often cynical or sceptical about the degree to which structural change will alter the nature of service delivery and its quality. Staff who see opportunities for their own career progression are more often enthusiastic and committed. But for senior managers trying to introduce change, it has been necessary to devise strategies (to do with training, preparation and incentives) to overcome some of the resistance (Dalley and Brown, 1988).

A second, and major, emerging issue has been the tension revealed between the principle of general management on the one hand and professional leadership on the other. It is a reflection of the wider impact of general management in the health service as a whole but comes into sharper relief at the sub-unit level because many more staff are involved – field staff as well as middle and front-line managers. Thus community nurses are having to adjust to the possibility of being managed directly by locality managers who may or may not be nurses; similarly, administrative and clerical staff or some of the professions allied to medicine are also being managed by locality managers not from their own professional background. Staff are being managed by a general manager and given professional advice and leadership from a senior professional designated as professional adviser. A clear distinction is having to be made between what constitutes the general management task and what remains part of the responsibility of professional leadership.

A third problem relates to the importance of acquiring accurate, up-to-date relevant information. Difficulties have been encountered in making the mix of hard and soft information accessible. Although Körner information requirements are intended to meet these needs, many districts have found difficulty in moving beyond routine data collection with little feedback to a method that collects and uses information sensitively and appropriately. The importance of having sound information is regarded as essential if the allocation of resources according to locality can proceed equitably.

A further issue is one which relates to the building of good relationships with other agencies. There is a body of both empirical and research evidence (SMAC/SNMAC, 1981; LHPC, 1981; Bruce, 1981; Dalley, 1989b) which demonstrates the problems involved in building interagency and interprofessional co-operation. In terms of locality management, the problems are particular. The essence of the locality approach is that it is geographically based. It focuses on the population of a defined geographical area. This may differ markedly from the approach of other agencies. Many local authorities now work to defined areas, but they may not necessarily be conterminous with health authority localities. The chief problem, however, is with GP practice populations; these are not usually geographically determined. A GP prizes the freedom to recruit patients from any area – in the name of patient freedom of choice. The GP feels constrained if the local health authority imposes boundaries, especially insofar as they relate to the community nursing services which are either attached or aligned to the practice. The benefits accruing to a locality perspective which the health authority sees are not necessarily recognized by the GPs within the same area. This has proved to be a difficult and sometimes intractable problem. Nevertheless, some progress is being made in some districts (Dalley, 1988).

One remaining major issue is the problem of evaluation. Making an effective evaluation of a complex process such as the introduction of a new management and service delivery system is fraught with difficulties. Many factors are involved: the effect of existing structures and the personnel occupying positions within them; the low morale existing after long periods of uncertainty; the impact of incomers with new, often contentious, ideas; the content of new plans; their time-tabling; outside influences beyond health authority control (local authorities, GPs, central government policies). Such factors all interact with each other; it is hard to distinguish the impact of one set of variables from another. The time factor is of crucial importance. 'Success', in terms of health outcomes (that is, a measurable change in the health status of a particular population within a decentralized unit), is likely to be slow to emerge (and immensely difficult to measure). Community units have had a short life so far and localities within them even shorter; comprehensive evaluation in so short a time is improbable.

FUTURE DEVELOPMENTS IN THE COMMUNITY HEALTH SERVICES

Most managers might argue that they need time to consolidate their achievements; the effective introduction of change is a slow process. However the health service has been subject to what appears to be a continuous process of change for more than a decade. The changes wrought by the 1982 reorganization and the introduction of general management in 1984–5 have had major consequences which have still not been fully absorbed. The experience of the community health services over the past five years demonstrates the radical effects that those changes have had. The changes instituted by the new general managers – such as decentralization – are still in the process of being put into place. While decisions have been made and changes introduced at the formal, structural level, movement in attitudes and culture has still to be secured.

Further changes, however, have now been proposed by central government. The White Paper 'Working for patients' (DoH, 1989b) published in February 1989 and the ensuing NHS and Community Care Act 1990 are remarkable for their failure to consider the position of the community health services. Nevertheless, they propose radical changes for the hospital sector and for GP services; these are bound to have repercussions for the community health services. The message of the legislation seems to be one of fragmentation and variation; hospitals and GPs are encouraged to become self-managing. One of the chief implications of this is that the coherent planning of services within defined areas and for defined populations will become more and more difficult. This must raise questions for community units. The rationale for the development of locality management has been based on the importance of accurately defining need in relation to geographically defined populations and tailoring services to meet such need. This requires coherent planning and integration of services across agency and professional boundaries. The probable outcome of the changes enacted in the legislation will be that such planning and integration becomes more and more unlikely. However, much resistance was voiced against the proposals: the extent to which they are successfully put into practice now that they are on the statute book remains to be seen.

4

Information use in effective community management

Margaret McArthur and Simon Stone

INTRODUCTION

Data collection is a task which looms large in the working lives of many community field staff. At the same time, community managers cast round desperately for information that will help them to make appropriate decisions. Surely the purpose of collecting data is all about providing just that information – or is it?

Too frequently information is not given sufficient priority by managers or field staff. There is a tendency, particularly amongst health care professionals, to challenge the accuracy and relevance of the information available, while at the same time duplicating data collection for their own purposes. Information has had a chequered history in the NHS because collection has always come before use, but there are many indications that this is changing.

During our time with the Management Advisory Service (MAS),[1] we worked with a number of community services on information-related issues. Such projects ranged from defining the information requirements of a health centre, to developing an information strategy for a Community Unit. In writing this chapter we have tried to communicate the practical lessons we have learned through working in the field, and at the same time to demonstrate the potential that exists for using information to assist community managers in their decision making.

So what do we mean by information? The word implies that those who receive it increase their knowledge in some way; con-

[1] The Management Advisory Service is a Charitable Trust which undertakes consultancy work within the health service on a non-profit making basis.

versely, if knowledge has not been increased, then it cannot be called information. A 20-page computer print-out, stiff with numerical data, cannot be called information unless the recipient has some understanding of what it conveys.

As the concept of information is not necessarily helpful while it remains abstract, it may be more useful to think about information in terms of the forms in which it may appear for a community manager. Four main categories can be identified:

1. **Bibliographic** The information to be gleaned from journal articles, reports, books. From published sources information may be obtained about the experience of other managers in developing community services, or in dealing with common problems. Material with a clinical focus may stimulate new approaches to service delivery, or provide a manager with enough knowledge to open up debate with professional staff about appropriate forms of care.

2. **Administrative** This category includes information contained in government circulars, in legislation such as the Health and Safety at Work or Education Acts. It also includes national, regional and local policies which shape the way in which services are planned and delivered. It comprises the rules within which managers must operate.

3. **Services and resources** This is not an easy group to categorize. It encompasses information about the local population, about the resources available for the provision of health services, about the way in which resources are used, the activity of services, their appropriateness, effectiveness and efficiency. Most health service information gathering has in the past focused on crude information on numbers of people seen or clinics held; this is now changing.

4. **Subjective** Information obtained through seeking the opinions of people, of service providers, of consumers or other interested parties. It is often tempting to disregard subjective information as somehow not as valid as the other categories (though all information is, to some extent, shaped by individual values and opinions). While care needs to be taken in how subjective information is obtained and used, it is an important ingredient of effective decision making, not least when used to corroborate other types of information.

Information may be obtained and presented through a variety of media, such as video, television and radio, in addition to the printed and spoken word. These more recently developed vehicles for information have a great potential for making it more accessible and for communicating it effectively.

This chapter largely focuses on the services and resources category. While, as we have demonstrated, this category represents only one aspect of the types of information essential to managers, it is the area where the most development is occurring, where changes in information technology are opening up new possibilities and where the greatest potential lies for helping managers to improve the delivery of services.

The approach we take in this chapter is, first of all, to think about the tasks facing community managers at all organizational levels within the current health service, and the relevance of information to these tasks. Secondly, we look at a variety of areas where developments are occurring, and at the potential of the types of information generated to inform the tasks of community managers. Finally we discuss the development of information strategies for community services, and offer some examples of ways in which information can help community managers now. While advances in computing have enabled many of the developments we examine to take place, we will not be looking at technological solutions in any detail, but concentrating on the information that can be delivered from them.

THE CURRENT CLIMATE

Over the last few years there have been a number of developments in the community health care environment which have affected the provision of information for management. Firstly, patterns of care have been changing. In line with national policy for the priority care groups, health authorities are increasingly planning for services to be delivered in community rather than institutional settings. Effective community-based health care relies on close working between health services, local authorities, non-statutory organizations, and informal carers and families. Multi-disciplinary working is espoused, particularly in mental health and elderly services. The White Paper 'Caring for People' (HMSO, 1989) gives new impetus for the provision of information about 'health' and 'social' care.

The dispersal of community services makes the task of gathering information about them more difficult. It is far easier to monitor services provided in a hospital by a limited range of professionals working for the same authority, than to know what is being provided to people in their own homes. The need for a range of professionals to share information about individual clients or about the resources available for providing care is complicated by the boundaries that tend to exist between professional groups and, moreover, between organizations.

The development of general management wthin health authorities following the NHS Management Inquiry (Griffiths, 1983) has been a further significant factor in changing the community health care environment. With general management has come a greater requirement for individual field staff and managers to be accountable for their activities and use of resources. There is an increasing concern to measure and improve the quantity and quality of services provided. The ideas contained in 'Caring for People' may change the responsibilities and nature of the agencies involved in providing community services, but they are unlikely to diminish this concern; more probably, better management information is likely to be crucial to their success.

Finally, there is the move on the part of many health and local authorities towards locality or patch management. The role of locality manager may carry with it a responsibility to develop services which are sensitive to local 'needs', for which purpose a range of information will be required about small geographical areas. This is in tune with a general concern, particularly from government, that health and welfare resources should increasingly be targeted at those whose needs are greatest.

These changes have been coming about at a time when computer technology is advancing rapidly from one year to the next. Until very recently, mainframe computers were the prime source of computing power for the average health authority. Now there is a far greater use of mini and micro-computers which have developed dramatically in processing speed and power, and have at the same time decreased relatively in cost.

Software is increasingly 'off-the-shelf' and both more user-friendly and more flexible to use than in the past. From being the province of initiates, computing power is becoming available to a far wider range of staff than before. This can ease the administrative tasks of operational staff, and at the same time provide managers with powerful tools for accessing and analysing resource and activity data. Rather than the cumbersome batch processing systems which used to prevail, data are increasingly input for primarily operational purposes, from where they are then immediately accessible to other users.

More use is also being made of communications networks, the most obvious example being the patient administration systems used in many health authorities, linking terminals within and between hospitals. There is a move also towards greater integration of different computer systems, to enable automatic transfer of information between them without the need for a paper stage. This at least limits the number of times that basic data such as patient identifiers have to be input, and at best allows powerful linking and analysis of information input through a variety of systems in different locations. Some hospitals are already achieving this level of integration (Faulkner, 1987; Lulham, 1988); the next step is to link community based systems. Resource management and the need for information upon which to base service contracts are already giving a greater stimulus to this process. Community based developments, however, are likely to be slower than those in hospitals.

As more computing power has been squeezed into smaller and smaller machines, portable and hand-held computers have become a practical option for field staff to carry, enabling data about what they do to be captured and transferred periodically onto a parent system for collation and analysis.

Trends such as these are enabling the development of computer-based systems which will increasingly help community managers to have access to information about service activity. Much of the impetus for development in community health services, however, has come from central directives such as the requirement to implement the Körner information requirements and child health systems, and the recent changes proposed in government White Papers ('Working for Patients', 'Promoting Better Health' and 'Caring for People') will help to keep up this momentum. With a range of developments being pursued it is perhaps timely to assess the ways in which these will generate information which can help community managers. In the following section we set out a framework for this assessment based on the kinds of tasks which managers face.

A FRAMEWORK FOR THINKING ABOUT INFORMATION FOR MANAGEMENT

There are legal requirements that dictate that certain types of information must be recorded, such as the treatment given to a patient. Certain information is required by higher authorities such as the Department of Health for monitoring health authorities, for which Performance Indicators are increasingly being used (DHSS, 1987). Other types of information may be collected for local reasons.

The collection of information is costly in terms of staff time and the equipment required. Judgements need to be made therefore as to how worthwhile it is to incur these costs. The prime justification for collecting information must be that it will be used in management or in clinical practice. The costs of collection are particularly an issue where the information collected is not providing any direct benefits for field staff in handling their caseloads, and is not derived automatically from operational activities.

The Information Working Party (Körner) set down some general principles to guide the approach used by health authorities when developing systems for capturing management information. In essence, these were that information should be:

1. accurate, relevant and timely;
2. derived as a by-product of operational data handling where possible;
3. used to inform management decisions.

Moreover, the Körner minimum data requirements themselves were merely to be a starting point upon which local managers could build their own information requirements, as appropriate to local needs and circumstances.

With the resources available to health care constrained, there has been limited expertise and technology available for implementation and it has been difficult for health authorities to follow these principles as closely as was intended.

It is often easier to focus attention on the collection of information before thinking about how it will help decision making. A preferable order is to consider first the managerial tasks to be performed.

Management tasks can generally be divided into three main areas:

1. **Direction** Setting the direction for a service; developing

objectives and planning services in line with the population needs identified.

2. **Co-ordination**   Ensuring that services are delivered on a day-to-day basis; matching resources to service requirements.
3. **Control**   Ensuring that services are operating efficiently and effectively, and that objectives, standards and the defined direction are being achieved.

Not every task will fall easily into any one of these categories, and the proportion of individual managers' time devoted to each area will depend on their position in the organization. A manager who is relating directly to a group of community nursing staff, for example, may devote more time to co-ordination tasks than a Community Unit general manager who spends a higher proportion of time on setting and monitoring the direction for the community services overall. While traditionally it is the co-ordination tasks that have been pursued at the expense of the other types, effective management relies on all three categories.

Figure 4.1 gives examples of tasks faced by community managers which illustrate each of these aspects of management. These tasks

---

Direction
To identify the needs of the local population and participate in the development of services and facilities sensitive to these.

Co-ordination
To manage community nursing and administrative support staff and to co-ordinate community medical service activity.

To develop effective policies, procedures and systems in order to achieve management objectives.

To develop effective local mechanisms to ensure the necessary liaison with other statutory and non-statutory agencies, with GPs and with the local community.

Control
To agree with the general manager the level and standards of the services to be provided, and to monitor these services to ensure their effectiveness, economy and efficiency.

Figure 4.1 Examples of the tasks of community managers.

have been drawn from job descriptions for community managers encountered when undertaking projects for community services.

DEVELOPMENTS IN MANAGEMENT INFORMATION

In this section we take a broad look at current health-related information developments and examine their potential to assist community managers. We use three main categories of information to discuss these developments:

1. Information about the general population and the environment in which they live;
2. Information about named individuals;
3. Information about specific services and resources available for health care.

There are points at which these groups overlap but they are sufficiently distinguished for our purpose. Within each category we provide an overview of the type of information provided by current initiatives and consider where developments appear to be leading.

Information about the general population

Community services are generally provided in non-hospital settings to people living in their own homes. To community service managers information about the population resident in the district is therefore crucial for planning the availability and distribution of resources.

The baseline for information about the population is the national census, carried out every ten years. It is largely on the basis of information obtained through the census that the population of any defined geographical area, such as a health authority or district council, is estimated and projected into the future. Its limitation, however, is that it is only available every ten years, and as the next census approaches, data from the last become increasingly out-of-date.

Since the 1981 census some interesting work has been done with the range of demographic and socio-economic information collected through the census. One important initiative has been the development of 'deprivation indicators' (Jarman, 1983) for every ward in the UK. These indicators allow estimates to be made of possible demand upon health and social services resources through comparison between different localities. They take into account not only the proportion of under fives and over 65s (who traditionally place high demands on community and primary services), but also other factors which have been linked with poor health status, such as unemployment, overcrowding and lack of household amenities (Black, 1980; Smith, 1988).

Many community managers are finding these indicators useful when considering how best to target scarce resources within their areas. The indicators have caused some controversy due to a concern that they reflect urban rather than rural deprivation. Care needs to be taken in using them in rural areas.

Likewise, late on in the census period factors such as 'gentrification' may alter the population of a small urban area, or new housing developments may bring in more young families. Any analysis will need to be treated with caution, and this is one area where the observations of field staff will be important when weighing up the relative needs of patches.

The Office of Population Censuses and Surveys (OPCS) undertakes a range of population surveys between national censuses. These often highlight interesting social and economic trends, and while not of much use in identifying specific needs in small areas may still suggest new approaches and comparators. The OPCS produces a newsletter for the NHS (OPCS, 1990) which describes current studies and highlights analyses which may be useful.

Market research companies also analyse census data. It is possible to buy population profiles for small areas from such companies (e.g. CACI), giving a wide range of socio-economic information, but not all of it is of interest to health and social services. Computer packages are available which make it easy to map different census variables in order to see trends between small areas more easily.

Local Authority Information Departments, particularly where they have adopted 'patch' based working in housing or social services, usually have high quality analyses of census and other data which they are prepared to share. The Structure Plans produced by County Councils which include details of housing plans and potential development areas can also prove a useful additional source of information about a locality which may help in planning future services.

Information about causes of death and patterns of morbidity and mortality can help to identify local problem areas to which community resources can be targeted. This type of information is derived originally from data about individual patient episodes or from death certificates. It is most readily available in aggregated form, though there is much untapped research potential in individual patient records. If higher perinatal mortality rates or deaths from coronary heart disease are discovered in a particular area this may mean, for example, that the objectives and priorities agreed with health visitors need to be different there from an area where the most pressing needs are among isolated elderly people.

It is often not possible to obtain statistically significant epidemiological data for areas smaller than a District Health Authority, because the numbers of cases involved are too small. It is worthwhile seeking advice from people trained in epidemiology (such as Consultants in Public Health Medicine) when gathering and interpreting this sort of information, and working with them when developing service plans. The annual report on the health of the population produced for each health authority by its Director of Public Health (as heralded in Circular EL(89)P/1) should increasingly prove to be an important source of information for the planning of community services, and the monitoring of their impact.

Information about the population in general and the environment in which they live can help managers of community services make decisions on the appropriate allocation of community resources between small geographical areas. There is no simple answer to how this should be done, although an example of how it might be approached is given at the end of the chapter. In addition to the types of information we have just been discussing, some knowledge of how and for whom resources are allocated at present is also necessary, which brings us to the second category of health-related information concerning named individuals.

Information about named individuals

Data are held on health-related computer systems about virtually every individual in the country. Some individuals will appear on a number of systems, whilst others may only be listed on their Family

Practitioner Committee register, depending on the contact they have had with health and welfare services.

Figure 4.2 illustrates the range of databases on which identifiable data may be held. The list is not exhaustive and not all systems listed are running in all areas of the United Kingdom at the time of writing. Nevertheless large quantities of data about individuals and the care they receive are now contained on computerized databases.

Körner Report 5 (DHSS, 1984) describes a minimum data set which should be collected about the activity of community-based nursing staff. Implementation of this report has resulted in the adoption by health authorities of systems such as Comcare, FIP, COM:ICS and others. Although some of these systems were initially

---

HEALTH SERVICE
Hospital
Patient Administration System (PAS)
(a) Patient Master Index
(b) Accident and Emergency System
(c) Inpatient Module
(d) Maternity Module
(e) Outpatient Module
(f) Waiting List Module

Pathology System
Radiology System
Pharmacy System

Paramedic Activity Systems
Ward Nursing System

Community
Child Health System
Mental Handicap Register

'Patient-centred' Community Nurse Activity System

Paramedic Activity Systems

FAMILY PRACTITIONER SERVICE
FHSA Register
Cervical Cytology call and recall
Breast Mammography call and recall
GPs' own systems

LOCAL AUTHORITY (SOCIAL SERVICES)
'At-risk' Register

Figure 4.2 Systems containing health-related identifiable data in relation to the organizations which manage them.

staff-based in that they recorded an individual's activity without linking it to the client, most now build a picture of the interventions that an individual client receives during an 'episode of care'. At the same time, the adoption of Child Health Systems by health authorities is increasingly providing a comprehensive picture of the interventions received by chldren and, to a limited degree, the effect of these interventions.

While many of the above systems were initially developed as stand-alone solutions, recent trends have been towards linking systems at the level of client identification, so that data can be combined, for example, about all aspects of a patient's stay in hospital. Clearly, moves towards resource management systems will accelerate this process (further discussion on this is contained in the section below on 'Moving towards a comprehensive and accessible information base').

In Figure 4.2 the various systems which contain health-related identifiable data have been shown in relation to the organizations which manage them. Organizational boundaries present many information problems, not least where community-based services are planned and delivered between a number of different agencies. When information about individuals is not shared between different carers, at best there is much duplication of data, and at worst clients suffer and resources are misdirected, because the left hand is unaware of what the right hand is doing. Several recent initiatives have begun to break down these boundaries, some examples of which are as follows

(1) In Oxfordshire District Health Authority a common Patient Index is now used for both hospital and community health systems.
(2) A major project conducted by the MAS with the Corporate Data Administration, the four health authorities in Devon and the local FPC, explored ways of managing screening for the county. Changes recommended included the development of a common screening system capable of managing call and recall for a variety of programmes, including child health, cervical cytology and breast mammography. The MAS further recommended that a single agency such as the FPC should co-ordinate and manage the delivery of all screening.
(3) Scottish Health Boards, which manage hospital, community

and General Practitioner services are developing 'community health indexes' for the populations they serve which are intended to link a range of primary, secondary and tertiary care systems.

(4)   An experiment sponsored by the Department of Health is currently underway in Exmouth to test the practicalities of using 'smart card' technology to enable the easy transfer of information about patients between the various agencies involved in their care. Plastic cards the size of a credit card, each containing a microprocessor, have been issued for approximately 8500 people, mostly children under five and the elderly. Whenever the individual visits their GP, the district general hospital or local community hospital, their dentist, or even the local chemist for a prescription, he/she presents the card which is read via a card reader and computer, and electronically updated as necessary. Each agency will be able to see what contact there has been with the others, and what the current position is.

The aim is not only to facilitate the sharing of basic information between the different agencies concerned to improve the care of the individual, but also to do so at a modest cost and under secure conditions. Each card is programmed so that only authorized users with the appropriate equipment can gain access to the information stored on it. If this experiment is successful we may see the use of card technology spread, particularly with the elderly and people with diabetes, where there are a number of different agencies involved in caring for an individual (Goldman, 1988).

There is indeed no legislative reason why systems carrying information about individuals should not be integrated and there are other examples of health, FPC and local authority cooperation at a local level which have developed to reduce the problems caused by these organizational boundaries.

Anxieties about confidentiality provide one of the main stumbling blocks to closer integration, as does the wide range of hardware and software used to support the various systems in use in health and welfare services. The development of the NHS Data Model and the definition of common communication standards are beginning to deal with the latter problem, whilst security methods which control access to data may help to make the confidentiality issue less of a concern.

Information about specific services and resources available for health care

Information about the resources available to meet the identified health needs of the community tends to be fragmented and partial. As the number of agencies involved in delivering health services increases, it is becoming increasingly important to maintain accurate and up-to-date information about the range of services available, from whatever source. While such information is of obvious value to planners and managers of community health services, it really needs to be accessible to referrers and providers of services so that clients can be offered the most appropriate response to their needs.

Sources of such information tend to follow organizational lines, with health, social services, family practitioner services and voluntary agencies maintaining records of the services they offer and some detail (frequently dated) about what other agencies provide. Some cross-agency initiatives have been developed in parts of the country; Help the Aged for instance have developed booklets for some areas which list a wide range of services for elderly people. East Dorset Health Authority in association with their local Social Services Department has developed a computerized database which encompasses a range of services for all client groups. Initiatives of this type are still, however, relatively uncommon.

When questioned, many field staff acknowledge that while they feel that they know about some of the services which are available to their clients, they tend to build a relationship with only a few possible alternatives and therefore refer in a circumscribed manner. It is also the case that staff do not always consider alternative ways of meeting a client's needs and continue to provide a service when other individuals or organizations might be more appropriate.

The thrust of Roy Griffiths' proposals for community care (Griffiths, 1988), resource management initiatives and, indeed, the recent White Papers, is towards the development of a wider range of services involving partnerships between the statutory, voluntary and private sectors. The provision of choice to clients and to service providers is also inherent in these initiatives. For these reasons it is clear that staff and clients should have ready access to a comprehensive directory of services and resources. Such a directory should ideally be computerized, allowing searches to be made using 'key words'. Entering, 'ELDERLY/LOCALITY X/ FOOT/ DISABLED for instance, would elicit a list of chiropodists, foot care assistants, etc., who offer a service in the locality, whose clinic is accessible to a disabled person, who treat elderly clients, how to refer to them, and possibly, how long their waiting list is. The client would, through such a system, be able to choose who to book with.

MOVING TOWARDS A COMPREHENSIVE AND ACCESSIBLE INFORMATION BASE

A common and justifiable complaint about many of the computer-based systems, which we have referred to above, is that whilst putting data in is relatively straightforward, producing anything more than the preset standard reports can be time-consuming, difficult and sometimes impossible. Recent developments in the use of fourth generation programming languages, which are specifically designed to allow easy and flexible access to data stored on computer should help to change this.

In the future, community staff themselves should be able to specify how they want to interrogate a database and to obtain timely and usable information from it. It should be borne in mind that there are always pitfalls in analysing and presenting data and that staff will need support from people with some knowledge of the way the data have been entered and the definitions in use, as well as of legitimate ways of manipulating it.

The heavy investment made by Community Units, both in systems and in staff development and training, means that whatever their limitations, existing systems will provide the basis for data collection and information production for some years to come. Indeed it can be argued that few authorities have yet exploited the power of their existing software and information base.

A more fundamental criticism of existing activity measuring systems is that they tend to provide little information about the purpose and outcome of contact between health professionals and the client. In this regard they have limited value as the basis for developing 'resource management' systems.

The central aim of resource management may be described as 'enabling the people who commit resources to make informed choices'. Resource management is both about devolving responsibility to the organizational level where resources are committed, and about providing accurate, relevant and timely information that will help the individual responsible to make better decisions. Effective resource management can be seen to rely on being able to link a range of information concerning:

1. Needs for services
2. Activity of staff
3. Alternative ways of meeting needs
4. Resources controlled by the authority
5. Other resources available including those controlled by statutory, voluntary and private agencies
6. The effectiveness (outcome) of services
7. The cost of services

Developing access to and easy links between these various elements of information may not seem to be a likely prospect in the near future, although a worthwhile state to aim for (see section below on 'Developing an information strategy'). But when it does become easier to obtain and link this sort of information, managers will have a more rational basis for decision making.

Well-integrated systems will not, however, take all the pain out of decision making; the subjective ingredient cannot be ignored. The preferences of individual clients, of carers, of local communities, opinions on the ethics of promoting certain services above others, the local political climate: all these subjective elements of information are needed to produce well-rounded decisions. If the objective information can be obtained with ease in the future, then perhaps managers will be able to expend more effort on obtaining the subjective information that will help them to formulate achievable plans, and to develop services which are responsive and appropriate to local needs.

DEVELOPING AN INFORMATION STRATEGY

We have demonstrated a range of different areas where information can assist community managers. We have also discussed developments which may in the future make it easier to obtain information that will help managers and field staff to identify needs and target resources accordingly. Careful planning will be needed to take advantage of these developments and others which will arise along the way.

Going through the process of developing a strategy for information is in itself a good way of clarifying problems and priorities. Strategies soon become out of date, so if they are to be of any use they must be living documents, frequently referred to and adjusted as circumstances change.

Each District Health Authority should have an information strategy of some sort, which may or may not be detailed enough for community purposes. If not, it may be productive to work through the information needs of the community in more detail and to check that these will be served. A district strategy will, however, act as a useful framework for developing a more detailed plan for community purposes, and should also demonstrate how the interface between community, hospital and DHA systems will operate.

There are a number of points which a strategy should cover. These can loosely be summed up by the questions: 'Where are we now?'; 'Where do we want to be?' and 'How do we get there?' In working with a community unit to develop a strategy for information (Hurst and Stone, 1988) we found certain ingredients of the strategy to be key: a definition of the principles which will underpin future developments, a 'vision' for the future, and a description of the various elements of that vision in practical terms. We will now describe these aspects of a strategy in more detail, using examples drawn from our work with the community unit.

Guiding principles

Defining guiding principles when developing a strategy will serve a number of purposes. Principles set out the constraints within which any plans must work. They provide a basis from which to develop detailed specifications and by the same token criteria to judge various options which may arise. Some principles will be broad and all encompassing:

1. Information plans must reflect and support strategic plans for service developments, such as the move towards less institutionally based care and the emphasis on targeting services towards 'at risk' groups.

2. Information plans should conform with extant policies on data protection and confidentiality.
3. Staff should be adequately prepared in terms of knowledge and skills to enable each stage of the strategy to be introduced successfully.

Other principles will be more specific and relate to different types of information, such as the provision of information for operational purposes, for planning or for monitoring. The following principle concerned monitoring:

4. Systems should allow field staff to input and obtain information about their performance and effectiveness, such as the balance of time spent on different activities or the outcome of different interventions.

In addition there will be principles which guide the detailed specification of systems. These may cover such areas as the presentation of information in graphical form to make it more immediately accessible to users, or the ease with which staff can gain access to systems and tailor their own reports.

The value of developing principles lies not only in their use for assessing alternatives but in the process of debate through which they are developed. Field staff may welcome the chance to participate in the discussions and may at the same time increase their understanding of information and its potential for use. Their input will help ensure that the principles are in tune with the way that community services operate.

The vision

The purpose of describing a 'vision' for the future is to make apparent to all whom the strategy concerns the end point that is being pursued. It should, therefore, be written in terms which conjure up as vividly as possible how future systems will appear to those using them, and what impact implementation of the strategy will have on consumers as well as field staff and managers. Figure 4.3 gives an indication of the range of benefits that different users should gain from implementation of one particular information strategy.

Such a vision will have to be brought into focus now and then

From the Consumer's perspective:
Will be able to request, confirm, modify and cancel appointments, electronically.

Will be able to make **informed** choices, with ready access to up-to-date information about the range and types of services available, where they are located, how effective they are, and how to gain access to them.

Will be able to request services, register with a GP, ascertain what particular services a GP offers, identify their local health visitor, the location of child health clinics, etc.

From the Field Staff's perspective:
Will have on-line access to a full range of information about their case-loads and, via hand-held devices, will carry information about their caseload and about services into the client's home.

Will have on-line access to a care planning module and the ability to record (and review) measures of outcome/effectiveness

Will be able to target their own time more effectively by an ability to plan tasks and to identify others involved in client's care.

Will be able to send and receive messages, referrals, etc. electronically.

From the Manager's perspective:
Will have frequently updated profile information about the population and about resources for the planning function.

More sensitive validated at-risk indicators will be available to aid decisions on where resources should be targeted.

Will have access to on-line resource utilization and activity measures.

Will have access to quality measures (e.g. waiting times by service, by facility and outcome/effectiveness indicators).

Will be able to identify shortfalls in skilled staff and to redeploy resources.

Will be able to identify the training needs of individuals and of groups of staff. They will have access to information about training opportunities and the ability to tailor local training initiatives to meet the defined needs of staff.

Will be able to link different data rapidly, to obtain more timely and sensitive indicators of performance and to develop 'what if' models for planning.

Figure 4.3 The vision

as developments in technology, changes in the organization of health care and other factors affect what is both possible and desirable. Again, it is a useful vehicle for broadening debate and encouraging the participation of those who will be affected by developments in information systems.

Elements of the vision

In order to allow practical plans to be developed for progressing towards the vision, its constituent parts need to be separated out and worked through in detail. We present some possible elements briefly in Figure 4.4 to demonstrate the range of areas where participants in the development of the strategy perceived the tasks of staff and managers could be helped by better and more easily available information. Many of these elements are termed 'directories', or 'systems'. This is to make it easier to understand what they are, and does not necessarily reflect how computerized data would need to be structured.

The heart of this array of future information systems will be the **Management Information System**. This will develop from existing financial systems by incorporating data from all the other operational systems. It will retain data sets from previous routine reports to allow comparisons over time. By allowing data to be imported from operational systems and combined in different ways, e.g. activity by population by cost, more sensitive management information will result. Additionally, data drawn from operational systems will be manipulated in different ways, particularly to assist with 'what if' modelling.

The **Population/Environmental Profile** will serve as a central system for collecting and aggregating data about the population served and sub-sets of the population. It will also provide a basic structure for collecting and aggregating data about the environment, at individual residence level, postcode level and at higher aggregations. Linked to this system will be the **Community Health Index**. This will contain a more comprehensive data set about individuals who have been, are, or are expected to be in contact with the service. It acts as a Community Master Patient Index (MPI) and by providing the link between community and hospital services will provide basic information about a client's medical and social

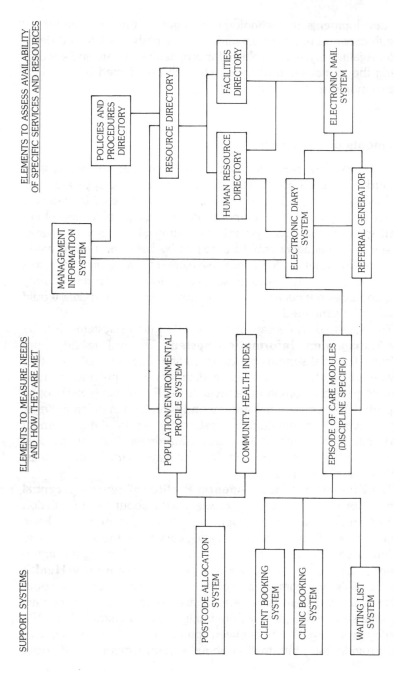

ELEMENTS TO ASSESS AVAILABILITY
OF SPECIFIC SERVICES AND RESOURCES

ELEMENTS TO MEASURE NEEDS
AND HOW THEY ARE MET

SUPPORT SYSTEMS

Figure 4.4 Elements of a comprehensive information system

history. Additionally it will contain a list of all staff in contact with a client.

Detailed information about each 'episode of care' will be held in discipline-specific **Patient Care Module(s)**. Each module will incorporate assessment data with a problem/needs list. For each identified problem or need, the desired outcome of intervention, planned action, a record of actual action and an evaluation of the degree of achievement of desired objective, will be recorded. To assist the costing of care the system will also collect data about non face-to-face client-based activity (telephone calls, case note and report writing, case conferences, sessions with carers and other health professionals). To assist them, staff will have access to an 'expert system', a database of problems, with a range of outcomes and actions, etc., designed to build up a comprehensive care plan for a client.

A range of support systems will be accessed via terminals by staff. A **Postcode System** will not only allocate postcodes to specified addresses, but will also store a range of data about the physical condition of residences and environmental factors about the immediate locality. Thus, in future, when a client moves into a new house, those risk factors which are related to accommodation will be automatically updated in their record.

Planned contacts between an individual member of staff and his/her clients, including location and purpose, will be recorded in advance by using the **Client Booking System**. This will reduce retrospective data collection, permit others to takeover planned care (or cancel booked contact) if necessary, provide information needed by the member of staff to plan their work and enable a client to contact the service and request, confirm, modify or cancel a planned contact. Similarly a **Clinic Booking System** will provide data about facility/service utilization, support booking of clients to a clinic, and/or to a specified time within a clinic, and support improved access by clients to services.

One of the current problems facing community services, how to measure demand for services, will be partially helped by the **Waiting List System**. This collects client-centred data about unmet demand for services and allows managers to highlight areas under pressure. It permits collection of data about demand for services which are not currently provided, by enabling staff to indicate that they would refer if the service existed, thus assisting service planning.

Information about the availability of services will be held in the computerized **Resources (Facilities and Services) Directory**. This will contain detail about all health service, local authority, voluntary agency and other services and facilities of interest to staff and clients (including health promotion and other general health-related services). Such a directory will list services and facilities (e.g. specified clinics) by type, availability, referral method, key contact, etc. The **Human Resource Directory** will supersede current personnel systems and provide a list of all staff employed or contracted to the Community Unit. It will act as a Community Unit Master Staff Index (MSI) and contain data about the skills, identified training needs, job history, reason for leaving, etc. of all staff. Linked to these two systems will be the **Policies and Procedures Directory**. This provides a cross-indexed directory of National, Regional, District, Unit and Locality policies and procedures. It also provides a cross-index directory to the range of State and local benefits, grants and other financial entitlements of potential relevance to clients and will include guidance on eligibility, how to apply for them and who to contact for further advice.

Clearly, underpinning many of the systems described above will be a network of terminals in every community staff base. Once such a network is in place, the creation of an **Electronic Mailing System** will be both feasible and highly cost-effective. Use of 'mailboxes' (with access restricted by password) will allow instant transmission of messages, referrals, test results, formal letters, etc. to an individual or group of specified individuals or a facility. The system will reduce the time spent trying to telephone another individual and provides the recipient with a dated and timed message. The network will permit rapid dissemination of hazard notices, and other crucial communications from Unit to staff and will confirm receipt.

In our 'vision' (Figure 4.3) we spoke about staff using hand-held devices to record and store data. Another benefit, in the future, of such equipment will be the ability they will offer to make an **Electronic Diary System** worthwhile. Such a system will enable all planned activity by an individual member of staff to be recorded, will allow identification of dates/times when specified individuals are available to meet and permit a client to identify a mutually convenient time for an appointment. Finally, we envisage the development of a **Referral Generator** which will allow potential recipient of referrals to define their information requirements by designing the referral form in terms of fields to be completed on screen. This will guide the referrer towards making more explicable and appropriate referrals by transferring data from the client record to referral form without re-entering data. The system would provide a hard copy of referral for transmission to non-computer-linked services and additionally would incorporate the date, time and referrer details into the client record.

A range of elements of a comprehensive information system are not listed here (for example, hospital activity systems) either because they are properly the province of some other agency, because they are already developed and are managed by another service, or because they clearly transcend organizational and geographical boundaries. Figure 4.2 lists a variety of these systems. The ability of community systems to link to them and transfer/share data when appropriate will be necessary if a comprehensive record of a client's health care is to be developed. Equally, other health authority systems such as the supplies system and the financial systems will contain data of value to the Unit in building a comprehensive information system for budgetary control and other management purposes.

We found in developing the Community Unit's information strategy that it was of considerable benefit to involve field staff in the process. From the staff themselves came a strong emphasis upon recording and analysing the effectiveness of different interventions, and a desire to have better information about the small populations they served. These are examples of areas which might not have been accorded such a priority by the strategy, had the development process been confined to managers and senior staff alone.

MAKING USE OF THE INFORMATION AVAILABLE NOW

It is always easy to defer using information until it is more available, more accurate, more up-to-date and so on, and to concentrate instead on developing bigger and better systems which will at some future date, specified or not, make it all possible. While this sort of procrastination is a natural part of human nature, it fails to recognize that through using the albeit imperfect information available now, the quality of that information can be improved. If field-level collectors of information see that others use it, and even better if they use or are monitored by the results themselves, then they will be more concerned to ensure that what goes into the system is accurate.

A culture in the organization which supports information use wll be equally necessary when information systems become more sophisticated. If this doesn't develop now, then all the sophistication and complex technology may be deployed in vain.

Because we feel it is important to foster this sort of culture from the outset we give some simple examples below of how community managers can use readily available information. We link these examples loosely to the tasks of community managers of which we gave examples in Figure 4.1.

TASK: *To identify the needs of the population and assist in the development of services and facilities sensitive to these.*

There is evidence that the needs of elderly people in the area are not being met, and that there are a number of recent instances where individuals have required hospital admission which might not have been necessary had they received some practical support and care in their own homes. As part of a wider strategy for the care of the elderly it is decided that more preventive community resources should be targeted towards elderly people in those areas of the district where their needs are particularly great. The following is just one approach that might be taken towards achieving this end in a rational manner.

Firstly, it is preferable to reallocate resources on the basis of achieving a clear objective. An objective might be to provide more face-to-face preventive support and advice to elderly people through increasing the proportion of time health visitors spend with those at risk to approximately 25% of their contact time. A sub-objective might be to target health visiting time spent with elderly people upon those living alone.

The expectation of pursuing such objectives might be that fewer elderly people are admitted to hospital because they have failed to care for themselves adequately.

Information about the general population provides at least three ways of looking at the relative needs of different geographical patches, each for example consisting of a group of wards. It provides an estimate of the total numbers of elderly people in each patch. It gives the numbers of elderly people living alone. Finally, the Jarman indicators allow comparison of the relative deprivation of each patch, which already includes the numbers of elderly people living alone but covers other important factors as well. This should be corroborated by subjective information from field staff working in the various patches, in case the census variables no longer reflect reality.

Information on the proportion of time health visitors are spending with different age groups may be available through a community information system such as FIP or COMCARE. By examining the census-based information on each patch and looking at the way in which health visitor time is being spent with the elderly at present (content of contacts as well as quantity), it becomes possible to form judgements as to how resources could be targeted better. The views of health visitors themselves about the needs in their own patches will need to be tapped. Finally, a combination of objective information and professional judgement will be needed as there is no magic formula for juggling the different types of information which feed into this sort of exercise.

The system which provided the initial information on how health visitors were spending their time should also provide information which will allow the changes in practice to be monitored. Information on the numbers of elderly people admitted to hospital, by reasons for admission, could show how far the expectations of achieving the overall objective were being met.

TASK: *To manage community nursing and administrative support staff and to co-ordinate community medical service activity.*

When 'direction' is defined for services, certain expectations about frequency and volume of services to be provided will be developed. A likely area for this to occur is the provision of Child Health Clinics staffed by authority-employed medical staff. Such clinics can, given consumer acceptance, provide a highly cost-effective method of monitoring the health of the child population in a locality. Additionally they provide a forum for conveying health promotion information and for ensuring that immunizations and vaccinations are offered to the population.

Current manual information systems provide sufficient information about the availability of nursing, clerical and medical staff to permit the manager to 'resource' clinics appropriately. When coupled with the opportunities that a computerized Child Health system offers for targeting invitations to attend (and reminders) at families who need encouragement to make use of the service, it should be possible to achieve a high utilization of current clinics, or to modify their frequency, timing or location, to improve utilization.

Co-ordination can thus be seen to be more than passively enabling services to be delivered; it also encompasses actively improving the effectiveness of services by identifying 'log jams' in the process of service delivery and taking action to resolve them.

TASK: *To agree with the general manager the level and standards of services to be provided and to monitor these services to ensure their effectiveness, economy and efficiency.*

In both of the foregoing examples the tasks of standard setting and monitoring are inherent. A crucial point about these activities, however, is that, having identified a failure to meet pre-set standards, the manager must be both willing and able to take action to remedy the situation.

In the first example, there would be little point in monitoring the activity of health visitors unless they could be persuaded or instructed to change their working practices, in this case to incorporate a higher proportion of visits to the elderly.

In the second example, unless there is a willingness to alter the times, frequency, location or role of a Child Health Clinic, knowing that some of them are under-utilized or busy but failing to attract those clients considered to be 'high risk', collecting information about their use is an expensive luxury.

In our breakdown of the management task we deliberately described the third element as 'control'. It is the use made of information which distinguishes a 'good' system from one which, however pretty the graphs it produces, merely places demands upon field staff to collect data without influencing service delivery.

CONCLUSION

Clemenceau once said that 'War is much too serious a thing to be left to the military'; we would contend that information, its collection, analysis and use, is too serious to be left to computer experts. A central role for an effective manager of community services is to develop and foster a culture within his/her organization which values and relies upon timely, accurate and relevant information to provide the basis for decision making. However exciting the next development in technology or software, real progress in using information depends upon a willingness to use what is already available. One indication of a successful information culture would be field staff themselves demanding improvements in systems rather than having 'improvements' thrust upon them.

Information is a crucial tool for effective community management. The complex mix of autonomous professionals, the range of organizations involved in community health care, the competing demands and priorities of the population and the ever increasing requirement to demonstrate efficient use of resources, all produce pressures and tensions for the community manager. Access to high quality information does not solve problems but, in many cases, it makes them manageable.

Part Two

Intersectoral Collaboration, Public Participation and Consumerism

5

Working with the voluntary sector

Rosemary Dun

> Most health authorities do not adequately recognise and support
> the contribution of voluntary organisations. Yet their strategies
> to promote good health and improve the quality of care, if
> they are to be effective, need to include work with voluntary
> organisations as an integral part of many services. (NAHA 1987)

This chapter will explore the problems and opportunities for joint
working between community health services and the voluntary
sector. The chapter will focus on the nature and organization of
the voluntary sector; the constraints under which voluntary organizations operate; the potential for joint working between community
services and voluntary organizations and the barriers and opportunities to joint working.

THE NATURE AND ORGANIZATION OF THE VOLUNTARY SECTOR

The voluntary sector represents organized forms of lay action and
is characterized by organizations with some formal structure (that
is, regular meetings, the keeping of minutes, having elected management or executive committees, and often with a written consti-
tution); that enjoy a high degree of autonomy; that are non-profit
making and often registered as a charity or limited company; that
may employ paid workers, a mixture of volunteers and paid workers, or rely solely on unpaid volunteers; and whose management
or executive committees work on a voluntary basis.

There is often confusion amongst those who do not have much

knowledge of the voluntary sector between volunteering and voluntary sector work. While volunteers might work with voluntary organizations and/or statutory bodies, they are not, of themselves, synonymous with the voluntary sector. The 'voluntary' part of voluntary organizations refers to the management and executive base – they always work on a voluntary basis receiving no fees other than expenses. Many of our largest institutions adopt similar practices, such as the NHS and local government, but they differ in that they are bound by statutory duties and are funded directly through taxation. The voluntary sector is autonomous. Each organization sets its own policies, aims and objectives. This accounts for its diversity.

According to Hatch (1984) the voluntary health sector provides 'a channel for three kinds of lay involvement . . . voluntary service, self-help and neighbourhood projects' as well as 'raising money for research, and services that rely on paid staff, like providing day care for addicts'. In the past, the role of the voluntary sector was usually regarded as that of applying pressure on the statutory sector to adopt services, change practices or listen to public opinion. Increasingly however, the boundaries are becoming blurred. The statutory sector is looking to set up its own voluntary sector initiatives. In addition the voluntary sector is being induced, to take on what, in the past, has been NHS provision.

These contemporary developments have widened the scope for mutual influence and learning between the voluntary and statutory sections. In terms of the consumer of health and social services, however, the voluntary sector is often seen to represent a choice or alternative to statutory services. For example, some people prefer non-NHS services, such as Brook Advisory Service, hospices, Relate (Marriage Guidance) or Crossroads Care Attendant Scheme, to their statutory equivalents.

Within the voluntary sector Community Health Initiatives (CHIs) have been an area of considerable development in recent years. Forerunners of CHIs were the six community health projects set up in the UK in 1977 by the Foundation for Alternatives. These projects were established as non-professional initiatives in neighbourhood health. All but one failed to survive beyond the first year of funding; Community Projects Foundaton (1988) and Scott-Samuel (1989) suggest that this might have been because they had not been rooted in the local community.

CHIs are primarily organized either around **geographical communities**, often neighbourhoods, e.g. Albany Health Project, Liverpool 8 Health Project, or around **communities of interest**, such as Health in Retirement–Fulham North, Avon Vietnamese Refugee Community Project, Lambeth Women and Children's Health Project. Many initiatives combine both approaches. Community action within these projects can range from and include any mixture of volunteering, self-help groups, campaigning, fundraising, social events, advice, counselling, advocacy, translating and training. What they have in common is that 'they aim to set up a process by which a community defines its own health needs, considers how those needs can be met and decides collectively on priorities for action' (CHIRU, 1987). CHIs are also based on common principles of taking a positive and broad view of health that goes beyond disease models; of aiming to reduce inequalities in health by addressing social, economic and environmental factors together with unequal access to health care; of wanting people to have better access to health information and resources, including information about the NHS and how it works. In addition, they want people to know how to lobby, organize and campaign; find ways of improving relationships between lay people and health professionals and to explore new ways of working in the community; increase self-confidence and to have more influence over health policies and allocation of resources (NCHR, 1988). According to Rosenthal (1983), an important characteristic of the Community Health Movement (CHM) is that it is based firmly outside the health professions. Essentially, the CHM at present mostly covers those projects that are voluntary sector based.

The emergence of an identifiable community health movement saw the establishment of two organizations – the London Community Health Resource in 1981 and the Community Health Initiatives Resource Unit in 1983. These were amalgamated in 1988 to form the National Community Health Resource (NCHR), which covers England, Scotland and Wales. NCHR is a voluntary organization, part of whose work is to support voluntary sector based CHIs.

Within the CHM there is an emergent debate as to whether CHIs are better situated within or outside the NHS in order to change or have an impact on policies. However, Morris (1984) stated that 'there is a strong case for authorities to view CHIs as something they should support but which should be outside, and seen to be outside their own immediate control'. The continuing autonomy of CHIs is arguably crucial to their success as it gives them freedom from bureaucratic and professional strictures. This gives them greater opportunities to cross boundaries, develop new ways of thinking and to bring people and organizations together in new relationships. These are prerequisites for social change and better health.

Self-help groups are another facet of the voluntary sector, that should be of concern to health managers. Self-help groups are often concerned with specific health problems. They may be linked to national networks such as MENCAP and MIND, and many cover chronic conditions, disabilities and interests, such as multiple sclerosis, caring for carers, schizophrenia and tranquillizer-dependency. Self-help groups can also arise from neighbourhood-based CHIs. These self-help groups and self-help activities of CHIs can be attractive to health professionals and managers as they provide additional services, support and promote mutual aid. As such they pose less of a challenge to professional viewpoints and can sometimes be viewed as a supplement, if not substitute for statutory provision.

HEALTH AUTHORITY FINANCING OF VOLUNTARY ORGANIZATIONS

Health authorities' funding of the voluntary sector amounts to just 0.01% of their total budget. This is made up from two main sources: joint finance and Section 64 funds. The level of grants varies between District Health Authorities, with a fifth of DHAs in 1984–5 making no grant or donation to voluntary organizations at all (NAHA, 1988). This represents a low level of investment in voluntary activity. Other sources of more short-term funding have been fairly easily obtained from Manpower Services Commission Community Programme or urban area funding from the Department of Environment. Many London-based DHAs have made much use of Inner City Partnership monies. This funding is usually available for 2 years with a 3 year maximum. These sources are now drying up and the MSC Community Programmes no longer exist.

Short-term funding leads to insecurity and makes planning difficult. Staff are often torn between loyalty to the project and the need to find more secure employment. Much staff time is spent trying to secure additional funding. This does not make for efficient organizations. However such arrangements can prove expedient to DHAs that do not take kindly to being challenged by local communities and are thereby given the means to let projects fade away as their funding runs out.

Community units with a real commitment to community development should provide what NAHA calls 'arms-length' financial support where funding is in general support of a CHI's objectives, is not controlled by the funding body – in this case the DHA – but is subject only to evaluation and periodic review of progress based on project objectives. Ideally, funding should be mainstream from the outset, but where the project is of a pilot nature, a commitment should be given to provide mainstream NHS funding if successful, according to the evaluation procedures agreed by the CHI and funding body. Nevertheless, this mainstream funding should ideally be given to the voluntary organization in the form of a grant rather than the project being located within district health structures and hierarchies. However, aspects of the CHI such as services or the way in which services are delivered could be assimilated into DHA services and practices if appropriate. NHS-based CHIs are a different matter and should be managed and funded by the DHA from the outset as part of an overall community development strategy.

A second method of funding would be via service contracts where the District Health Authority contracts out or buys in services. But this is a delicate relationship. Many in the voluntary sector do not see the role of the sector to act as a substitute for statutory provision nor to enable cuts in services. They see their role to be to pioneer services that, if relevant, are then taken on by statutory bodies. What the voluntary sector can often do is to provide services in a more flexible and acceptable way that meets individual and collective client needs, such as care attendant schemes, and independent living schemes, combining flexible packages of housing and personal care.

THE POTENTIAL AND CONSTRAINTS FOR JOINT WORKING

The State has a duty to meet the health needs of its populations and to consult with communities regarding those needs. But the State cannot meet need that is unrecognized. This reality arguably underlines the reluctance of the NHS to enquire about need, for fear that the floodgates of demand are opened. A dilemma then has been how to gauge need without necessarily having to meet all demands. This has led to many debates as to what is a 'need' and what is a 'demand'. CHIs, on the other hand, having no statutory obligation to meet unearthed need themselves, are free to explore this terrain. Indeed, it could be argued that CHIs themselves are a response to the failure of the NHS to meet need. As such they can provide invaluable information to community units seeking to address this issue. What CHIs do not do is to prioritize need. They have seen their role as being to lobby the NHS to meet demand – not to juggle financial and other restrictions. But, the State is there to provide a service and should be accountable to citizens who pay for that service through taxation. Therefore, citizens should be involved in decision making, regarding priorities, in partnership with health experts and managers. CHIs, as a form of lay representation, could provide one route. The NHS is not democratically accountable and has therefore not been subject to lay involvement; this could be said to be a major factor of the dominance of medical models and an NHS that is often criticized for serving professionals' needs rather than those of patients and populations.

Nevertheless, the reality is not straightforward. The NHS is a complex organization, reflecting many cultural conflicts and needs. There are open and hidden agendas contained wthin the question 'Why should community units seek to work with community health initiatives, and vice versa?'. The answer will depend very much on who is setting the agenda, their general approach and what they want. Reasons could be based on any combination of the following at any given time:

- to develop care by the community
- to get 'closer to the consumer'
- to find out what consumers/public want
- as a response to the growing popularity of Health For All and Healthy Cities Projects
- to influence lifestyle/behaviour amongst populations
- to identify markets/areas for targeting resources
- to make cuts in own services by transferring or contracting out services to voluntary and informal sectors

- to enable the monitoring of service provision by local communities
- to identify and/or develop constituencies to which to be accountable and with which to consult
- to develop formal/informal partnerships
- to ease early discharge policies and the decanting of patients from institutions to communities
- to gain consensus for policy and plans
- to tap resources, avoid duplication and plug gaps
- to promote the use of unpaid labour/volunteers
- to enable workers to work more flexibly with a resultant increase in staff morale
- to access local information
- to join forces with existing local action
- to advance the health of local populations
- to develop skills and learning together
- to promote and support self-help and individualism
- to set up processes for regular dialogue
- to develop local networks
- to provide support to local self-help groups
- to communicate DHA plans, priorities and policies
- to free resources in order to develop small community care units, e.g. group homes/residential units
- health authorities, as funding bodies, have a statutory duty to ensure money is spent in appropriate ways

Community units are being encouraged to make contact with their communities, to identify local need, to provide more flexible, responsive and appropriate services, and to promote community participation. The Griffiths report (1983) stated that 'a great deal of importance is attached to ensuring that the views of the community at all levels are taken into account in any decision'. A danger, however, is that making contact with CHIs might be viewed as *the* answer. But, CHIs are only part of the community. Furthermore, CHIs are direct responses to expressed need and few see their role as to monitor and meet the latent needs of neighbourhoods or the communities they serve.

WHY SHOULD COMMUNITY HEALTH INITIATIVES WORK WITH COMMUNITY UNITS?

A variety of reasons can be postulated for CHIs wanting to work with community units. These include:

- to gain funding
- to access expertise and information on health and on services
- to gain access to resources such as buildings, equipment
- to impact on health planning and services
- to enter into dialogue in order to express local need and demands
- to obtain appropriate and accessible services delivered in the ways that people want
- to access a route to effect change in health policy
- to forge working relationships/joint practices with front-line staff
- to gain recognition and increase status
- to gain power
- to give voice to local views

CHIs probably do not want much from health authorities. If anything they are concerned about the dangers of colonization of the CHM by the NHS. CHIs also tend to have low expectations, as past experiences have often seen their exploitation. They are wary that they might be viewed as an 'easy option' by community units that are under-resourced. What CHIs do want is funding. Typically they are grossly under-resourced. CHIs seek power in order to change or influence health policy. Financing not only supports the work of CHIs but also represents a fundamental devolution of power from the NHS to local communities.

The culture of the NHS is so strong that many CHIs can feel oppressed in collaboration exercises, and an atmosphere of suspicion, even hostility, is likely to prevail. Generally, there is a lack of understanding within the NHS of the voluntary sector. When many NHS people think of the voluntary sector they think of the volunteers that they have seen in a hospital setting, of the WRVS or League of Friends, or of the larger well known organizations such as MIND and Age Concern. They are relatively unaware of the diversity of the voluntary sector, the different **types** of organizations, and that although organizations are voluntary, they are not 'amateur'. This is largely due to the fact that until recently community care was mainly undertaken by local authorities. As a consequence, local authorities are a rich source of knowledge and expertise for health authorities seeking to work with the voluntary sector.

Conflict and ignorance are likely to mar collaboration unless acknowledged. Community participation and collaboration between the NHS and voluntary sector are often represented in cosy terms – the reality can come as a surprise that defeats partnerships. However, 'this [conflict] can be healthy if openly acknowledged and contained within clear and agreed objectives based on open negotiation. Healthy conflict can produce innovation, unhealthy conflict the adoption of polarised positions' (Dun, 1989).

It is essential that joint working between community units and CHIs is supported by 'those at the top as well as those at operational level' (NAHA, 1988) in order to be effective; lack of commitment at health authority member and senior management level has led to the demise of many CHIs, as partnerships can otherwise be too reliant on individuals who might leave, or on changing resource priorities.

A MIXED ECONOMY AND THE PLURALITY OF WELFARE

The NHS is looking more to 'mixed economy' solutions that fit the plural nature of welfare. This can provide many opportunities for community unit managers and for locality and neighbourhood managers, (if budgets are devolved to their level), to seek more flexible service and financial solutions to multiple needs and problems. A manager might then be able to view each client as someone with a mixture of needs to be met rather than trying to fit those needs to the services that the community unit manager already has. With devolved services and budgets a manager could obtain sufficient local knowledge and have the financial freedom to tailor local services – whether from statutory, voluntary, informal or commercial sectors – to fit needs. This might include the buying-in of services from the voluntary or commercial sector, based on suitable service contracts. East Sussex Social Services Department has developed a computer package for this purpose; it enables area and patch-based managers to plan, forecast and manage budgets and services for overall areas and client groups, as well as being able to access information on individual clients. Such a database could be used in the preparation of area health profiles.

A further option available to managers has seen the setting up of voluntary organizations in order to develop 'care in the community' housing and support packages, or the use of existing voluntary organizations, or the use of their own or local authority housing to house volunteers, organized by volunteer organizers, in order to provide more flexible independent living schemes for people with physical disabilities wishing to live alone.

Further benefits for community units in working with CHIs would be that CHIs can offer a balance to individualistic and medical models of health. They can foster innovation, free from the constraints of a large State bureaucracy. At their best, they can pinpoint ways to flexible and non-stigmatizing methods of planning and of delivering services. They can enable more appropriate and relevant data about people's health to be collected; they can cross organizational boundaries, perceive new ways of working, and bring people and organizatons together in new relationships via mechanisms such as management committees, forums and alliances. Many groups undertake local political activity in the form of campaigning for better or more appropriate services and for greater say in health policy and planning.

PITFALLS

Community unit managers are under pressure to produce quick results and could view CHIs as providing a number of 'easy' options; but, community development takes time and is more effective if it can build on small, achievable targets. The mismatch between lay/professional and CHI/NHS perceptions can lead to a dislocation in expectations. CHIs, and in particular those funded within or by the NHS, can be expected to do too much, too soon, and have too generalized aims; this in turn can leave the community health worker(s) faced with difficulties of focus on achievable objectives.

Community health workers tend to be junior in status and lowly graded in salary terms. In a status-bound hierarchy such as the NHS, they can find themselves with insufficient status to work with senior officers, doctors and nurses, let alone achieve often 'high-flown' tasks. NHS-based community health workers often lack health authority recognition and support. Thus pushed to the margins and even outside of the NHS, CHIs and community health workers are easly 'dumped' by managers if they become too challenging or if trends and priorities change. CHIs need to be clearly either within or without the NHS rather than straddling both camps.

Voluntary organizations, and in particular large self-help groups such as MIND and MENCAP, can be seen as a way of substituting for statutory services, providing community care on the cheap, or plugging gaps in service provision.

The involvement of voluntary organizations that represent 'minority' viewpoints can be viewed by some health authority managers and planners as addressing their equal opportunities policies. However, this route will not of itself address institutionalized racism, sexism and other discriminatory practices and attitudes – this can even be obstructive if not viewed as part of a more total process. Similar marginalization can lead to CHIs and other voluntary organizations being loaded by the health authority with total responsibility for the representation of 'their' community. This often happens at the level of expectation, without open discussion and without any increase in resources to CHIs, that are frequently single worker projects. A consequence is that subsequent overloading leads to inefficiency which then leads to funding being withdrawn with resulting bad experiences on both sides (McNaught, 1987).

Making contact and partnerships with the voluntary sector and CHIs will not provide full community participation and representation in itself. Working with CHIs is only one form of community participation. Health authorities need to identify their population mix and adopt robust equal opportunities/policies and practices that go beyond sex and race; they must also develop representation that reflects population mixes and needs. Where necessary, positive discrimination and active measures will be necessary to ensure the involvement of traditionally under-represented groups, such as people with physical and mental disabilities, carers, women with children, women, black and ethnic minority communities, unemployed people, gay and lesbian people, homeless people and homeless families, rootless people and travellers. CHIs cannot be expected to present comprehensive pictures of need in communities. They respond to expressed need rooted in the here and now and based on where, and the time of day, that community health workers work. CHIs are concerned with immediate and localized issues such as bad housing, social isolation, lack of child-care provision, lack of home helps/care assistance and will not necessarily relate these to more centralized issues such as lead pollution, industrial health issues and food irradiation, unless these become of more personal importance to the people involved in such collective health action. Nevertheless they are a valuable source of local knowledge, and barometer of local health opinion, but are not the sole indicators of need.

CHIs can represent collective and public responses to health that in turn can threaten the individual and private responses represented by medical viewpoints. Health authorities and health professionals have responded in the past by attempting to colonize CHIs in order to bring them within the safe confines of the NHS. This threat has fuelled a wariness on the part of CHIs of becoming involved with the NHS. Moreover, CHIs need the opportunity to develop their own strategies and solutions as a counterbalance to NHS professional and medical models. Indeed, the symbiotic relationship between the voluntary sector and the NHS is essential to development – especially for the NHS.

Further threats to CHI autonomy can be issued through funding, which can be abused as a form of political sanction. Some CHIs might find their self-help, but not their campaigning, activities funded, and some can experience the withdrawal of funding on failure to comply with explicit or implicit conditions. Funding should be on an 'arms-length' or contractual basis.

OPPORTUNITIES FOR JOINT WORKING: SOME EXAMPLES

It is currently the norm for health authorities to have no systematic policy towards voluntary organisations, to give only very modest financial and other support despite having the necessary powers, and to make no serious efforts to involve voluntary organisations in planning. Indeed, health authority officials and health professionals seem frequently to have a limited understanding of what voluntary organisations are, let alone know how to work with them. (NAHA, 1987)

As already outlined, working with the voluntary sector is not an easy or cheap option but the rewards can be many for community unit managers. However, in order to be effective, strategies and clear working practices need to be developed. To dabble is to risk the chance of a bad experience militating against future attempts at partnerships on both sides. Evaluation is also important as this ensures that lessons are learned by both sides and enables development to continue in spite of, and sometimes because of failure. What is needed are practices that will acknowledge, recognize and, hopefully, forestall any pitfalls.

Community units can find the voluntary sector fragmented and therefore difficult to engage in partnership. Managers often do not know where to start or how. Major reorganizations are not necessary and often just starting enables partnerships to grow. Nevertheless, a general, and where possible, stated commitment can demonstrate a will, and promote the way, as it engenders confidence on both sides and ensures that participants know where they stand. This section will explore some ideas and approaches for NHS community units which seek to work with the voluntary sector and CHIs in particular.

CURRENT STATE OF PLAY

As stated previously there are many reasons why community units might seek to work with the voluntary sector and CHIs in particular. All these forms of partnerships have their place, but my view is that the role of the voluntary sector remains essentially a passive one and the partnership is therefore unequal. Even patient participation and user groups serve only in an advisory capacity, allowing plenty of room for professionals and managers to filter opinions that only serve their own plans and purposes. There is little if any involvement in decision making.

Community units working with CHIs is fairly new. This is partly because the role of CHIs is primarily one of health promotion whereas the community unit's is to provide services and 'prevent' sickness; partly because CHIs challenge medical models and professional viewpoints; and partly because CHIs often have little need, beyond seeking funding, to engage with community units. Their broader definitions of what affects health tends to lead them to make alliances with other local voluntary sector organizations, with local authorities, and to seek to influence and work with local health workers and GPs directly.

At present, the voluntary sector's representation on policy making bodies is marginal. A typical situation can be the presence of one voluntary sector representative on a steering group which is packed with professionals. 'Official' voluntary sector representation is essentially limited to three representatives on Joint Consultative Committees, (JCCs), a CHC representative with observer status on the health authority, and often no representation on Joint Care Planning Teams and Client Care Planning Teams. The whole voluntary sector is often assumed, by health authorities, to be represented by one organization such as MIND or Age Concern. Health authorities, too, frequently wheel out the same 'community representatives' when they feel that they should have someone from the voluntary sector along. This raises questions as to who these people represent and to whom they are accountable. Often workers in CHIs complain that they are burdened constantly by health authority assumptions that they alone represent their 'constituencies' (an example being an Asian worker for an Asian health project who was often the only person called by the District Health Authority to represent her community and was invited to so many committees and working groups that her groundwork as a single worker covering a whole borough was suffering).

In the meantime, community unit managers are being instructed to ensure that they provide the services that people want and need, to decentralize to localities and neighbourhoods, to provide more accessible services, to get 'closer to the consumer', to increase effeciency and cost effectiveness, to promote mixed economy solutions and income generation schemes, and to develop integrated care systems between all sectors. In conjunction with this is an international call from World Health Organization for greater community participation, intersectoral collaboration, and the achievement of Health For All by the Year 2000 targets.

In the past District Health Authority community provision has been centralized and based on medical definitions. General management is leading to increasingly decentralized systems which themselves are opening up possibilities for health authorities to become more accessible and flexible. Benefits are not only for local communities but also for those local primary/community workers who feel dislocated from decision-making processes, unable to change the way they work, and powerless to affect people's health in the face of socio-economic and environmental factors and often incomprehensible and obstructive NHS hierarchies. In the past those health workers have been less likely to forge links with local

CHIs as they felt easily threatened, and frequently retreated to entrenched status-bound positions.

CHIs and community units are likely to have aims and objectives that are in conflict. Often only the positive sides of such partnerships are emphasized that leave participants unprepared for any conflicts imposed by different cultural bases, conflicting demands on limited resources, and the differing perceptions of lay and professional people. Health authorities might not be open about the constraints they have to deal with. The voluntary sector has also traditionally taken an oppositional stance, this means that they frequently do not fully understand the organizational strictures under which many professionals and managers in State bureaucracies work. Attempts at collaboration can fail due to lack of openness and skill in negotiating on both sides of a partnership, whereas agreed aims can contain such conflict and provide common goals. Clear structures are needed in all partnerships whether in setting the terms of reference for a forum or working party, whether agreeing aims of a newly formed voluntary organization, drawing up service contracts, or setting up procedures for accountability and participation in decision making (e.g. locality planning groups, local advisory groups, patient participation groups, user participation groups). Voluntary organizations also need to understand and have information on the structure of the health service.

Health authorities need to have flexible arrangements in order to cope with the non-uniformity of the voluntary sector. Appropriate DHA staff need to develop working relationships with umbrella voluntary organizations in their areas (e.g. borough disability organizations, Councils for Voluntary Service or Rural Community Councils). Positive steps should be taken by DHAs to identify those voluntary organizations which have a specific interest in its services or in health issues generally and to understand their aims and expectations. They should not, however, expect any one 'body' to represent the entire voluntary sector, although umbrella organizations can provide a fuller form of representation. Voluntary organizations, in turn, need to recognize that DHAs face problems in seeking to relate to a diverse and relatively unco-ordinated voluntary sector, and be prepared to work together through umbrella bodies such as RCCs, CVSs, or other forums, to enable representative input. It is also important that DHAs take a wider view of the voluntary sector that extends beyond service providers to include groups representing people, e.g. tenants and residents associations, and self-help groups that form around problems related to illness, disability and carers. Also those groups campaigning for better services, more say, health rights, advocacy, advice and information giving, and which are constructive critics of service providers or promoters of innovation are regarded by many as being vital in helping to make the best of public funds. They also merit funding and other forms of support.

The agenda for debate should not be dominated by health authorities. Dialogue is a two-way process and not simply asking for comments on a health authority's ten year plan. Health authorities must be prepared for their programmes and priorities to be challenged, and local communities, together with the voluntary sector, need better, clearer and more accessible information from DHAs in order to participate fully. Some examples of joint working opportunities follow.

(i) Information

Many health authorities are turning to the voluntary sector and CHIs in particular to furnish them with information regarding local need. But, the voluntary sector does not have the resources or the statutory duty to carry out such a function. It is unlikely that it can do anything other than provide 'grassroots' knowledge regarding its own client groups and communities. It cannot be expected to provide an overall picture. It can, however, provide much information regarding the appropriateness of services and pinpoint possible gaps or overlaps in provision.

On the other hand, the health authority itself has much information regarding its populations, i.e. socio-economic and demographic as well as epidemiological, health indices and service indicators. Health authorities can build up profiles of district, localities, neighbourhoods and even ward and enumeration district data using existing information or linking with local authority information. Collaboration with Family Practitioner Committees can provide data relating to primary health services. Thus, information can be provided on a district basis and can be used in local planning in localities, neighbourhoods and patches.

Local health forums, community health workers and primary care workers working in community development ways could access such centralized information to enable the building up of local health profiles and community maps. These can be linked in with local voluntary sector directories denoting local activity. Much information is collected simply because it always has been; the involvement of the voluntary sector in decisions, such as what information to collect and how to disseminate it, will enable information systems to be more appropriate and sensitive.

To be fully effective information should not only be available for general managers and planners. Local communities and primary workers will need information from central databases that is usable and in accessible forms and health authorities need to communicate plans, priorities and policies for local consultation; this should combine with the collection of information from local to central bases, as well as local demands and expressions of need. Information gathering and dissemination should involve the participation of local fieldworkers and local voluntary organizations, including CHIs. Information should be fed back to local populations with some form of lay evaluation and monitoring of the information being collected and disseminated.

(ii) Community development approach

Some health authorities are adopting a community development approach to health and as such are aligning themselves with many of the principles of the Community Health Movement and CHIs. Parkside Health Authority and West Lambeth Health Authority have made moves to develop such an approach through proposals from a health promotion group (Farrant, 1986), the adoption of community development and groupwork in health visiting practices (Drennan, 1985), and a link with 'going local' (Dun, 1987). Riverside Health Authority has also adopted the WHO Health For All principles.

In essence, a community development approach to health and health services describes a process whereby health professionals have regard to local community health needs and involve local communities, wherever possible, in all aspects of their work. It also involves health professionals working with and sometimes initiating local groups in order to assist local communities to become more involved in their health and health decisions and to give voice to their needs. A community development approach usually involves the establishment of local community health worker posts. It also involves the putting into practice of CHM and Health For All principles by health authorities.

A community development approach calls for the percolation of these principles through all levels and, in particular, the adoption of local strategies. It requires health workers, managers and planners to work in different ways and in equal partnerships with local communities. The adoption of this approach can herald the coming together of the cultures of the NHS and the Community Health Movement.

How then is this community development approach put into practice? It takes time and clear principles, aims and objectives, in order to maintain a sense of direction in what Bayley *et al.* (1987) describe as 'the hard slog of turning . . . theory into practice'. Health authorities should develop a community development strategy and statement of intent. This can serve to validate and give permission to NHS community health workers to work in a community development way as well as demonstrating commitment to working with the voluntary sector and CHIs. In turn, this can do much to allay suspicions and enable everyone to know where they stand. This has been an important factor in the success of CHIs such as the Bristol Inner City Health Project. The Manager of the community sub-unit of the Bristol and Weston Health Authority made a written 'Statement of Commitment' in November 1987 concerning the involvement of community representation in the work of the Bristol Inner City Health Project (an NHS-initiated CHI), in order to allay the 'legacy of mistrust and suspicion towards the health authority'. Indeed, such a statement might have helped a doomed community participation exercise around a health centre in South London where a community physician, finding that he had no support from the then District Management Team and Health Authority members, was forced to let down a whole community that wished to be directly involved in the design, planning and running of the centre. Nine years on, local community groups are still suspicious of District Health Authority intentions.

As well as investment in time this approach demands investment in training. Some health authorities may go for the development of health visitors with community development roles, who then work with local groups, or as members of local teams working with groups, or work to promote the establishment of self-help groups (Drennan, 1988). Health authorities may also develop community health workers based on decentralized geographical areas such as localities or neighbourhoods; such CHWs should be employed by those health authorities, and be responsible to a senior officer with a district-wide role of community development. Community health worker briefs should be to develop community health profiles, support and initiate CHIs and self-help groups and activity, and be locally accountable to a locality or neighbourhood health forum for local priorities. Other CHWs might be facility based, i.e. on a health centre, and employed to make links with local communities in their catchment area, together with developing local initiatives and groups whilst being accountable to facility-based local advisory groups (as in West Lambeth Health Authority), or to a centre advisory group (as the Link Worker at Lambeth Community Care Centre), or to user participation groups. A further option could be the initiation by health authorities of CHI and CHW posts that are independently funded and within the voluntary sector.

These posts, and especially NHS-based CHIs and community health workers, are fairly new, and much confusion has arisen regarding issues of management, accountability, funding and support (Dun, 1987). Many NHS-based CHIs are being set up on short-term bases with 'soft' funding, vague and too generalized job descriptions, and a reluctance on the part of NHS management to – as they see it – relinquish control to local communities. These community health workers are left with no real identity, being neither part of the NHS nor the voluntary sector; they often have no authority in the absence of clear commitment to community development from the health authority, and experience conflicts of loyalty. The short-term nature of their funding, together with pressure to produce often unrealistic results, conflicts with the fact that community development takes time and there are no sort cuts. They are also easily cut, can be viewed as a 'luxury', and are thereby vulnerable. Nevertheless, benefits for community managers in adopting a community development approach can be many, not least the development of a community perspective and broader definitions of health being internalized by NHS workers to the extent that it becomes integral to their everyday work instead of something extra and distinct. Thus workers will not 'just focus on individual clients and their networks, but also on particular groups

. . . within their area. They (will) now call upon a range of community based resources and work "within the community" ' (Bayley et al., 1987).

Some health authorities, such as West Lambeth, are developing in a rather *ad hoc* manner, having no 'officially' approved community development strategy or statement of intent; others are developing a strategy in line with localization strategies (such as Bristol and Weston, Exeter, North Manchester and Islington).

At the heart of community development is enabling local communities to identify and articulate their health needs and to promote collective action around health issues, as well as building the self-confidence to be able to do so. Examples of possible solutions are: the establishment of an action project that produces an access survey of local health clinics, centres and doctors' surgeries and then campaigns for changes; the involvement by the local community in the design and running of a local community hospital (Lambeth Community Care Centre, Wilce, 1988); obtaining funding and setting up of a care attendant scheme; lobbying the council and gaining a community flat where a crêche can be run and classes arranged on health matters for residents of the local estate, with support from health professionals and voluntary sector workers, as well as talks on homeopathy and alternative health; and the establishment of a partnership between a local GP, local health visitors and local voluntary activity to form a homelessness project concerned with health, housing and child welfare (Bayswater Homeless Project).

(iii) The joint planning process and voluntary sector forums

The voluntary sector has access to joint planning activities between health and local authorities via Joint Consultative Committees (JCCs). JCCs consist of District Health Authority members, local authority members, one or two family practitioner members and three voluntary sector representatives. The voluntary sector representatives are chosen every four years by an electoral process. The role of the JCC is to plan and propose collaborative work across agencies and to decide how Joint Finance funding can best be used to meet community care needs for the District. JCCs also have access to all health authority minutes.

JCCs are advised, and plans and proposals are prepared, by the Joint Care Planning Teams (JCPT) sometimes called 'Senior Officer Support Teams', which also service the JCCs. Client Care Planning Teams (CCPT) are composed of officers at practitioner level of health and local authorities and are usually based on client or priority groups such as the elderly, mentally handicapped or mental health. Their primary role is to review needs and services for these client/priority groups in the District and to report to the JCPT who will decide district-wide priorities across client groups.

It is common for voluntary organizations to be invited to participate at CCPT level (as in Birmingham, Bradford, Manchester, Tameside and Glossop) but not at JCPT level. There is therefore a break in the chain of voluntary sector involvement in 'the joint planning process'. Also, JCC voluntary sector representatives are at a disadvantage as they are not briefed or serviced by senior officers attending JCPTs, unlike health and local authority members. In some areas the voluntary sector has successfully gained a place on the JCPT (as in Avon, Birmingham, Coventry, Riverside, Islington and Oxford). Some health authorities seek voluntary sector representation through the involvement of CHCs only, but this will not do. CHCs are not representative, and although 'independent consumer watchdogs' they are not part of the voluntary sector: they are NHS based.

Community unit managers could improve voluntary sector involvement in joint planning by ensuring at least one place for a voluntary sector representative on the JCPT. The next stage would be to approach the appropriate CSV or RCC or other umbrella organization and ask for their help in setting up a voluntary sector forum on health that could then provide the constituency, elect a representative to the JCPT, and be actively involved in District Health Authority policy-making regarding care in the community, thus ensuring a reporting backwards and forwards process. The forum could also provide the support needed for the often daunting task faced by a voluntary sector representative seeking to participate in a group of professionals. Such a forum should also include as members the CCPT and JCC representatives, thus enabling continuity. The second thing that community unit managers of DHAs could ensure would be a room where the voluntary sector JCPT and JCC representatives could meet before a JCC meeting; most DHA and local authority members have a similar facility. It would also be fortuitous if CCPT, JCPT and JCC voluntary sector representatives met regularly to decide their own agendas, objectives and priorities. A third requirement would be funding for administrative support for such a voluntary sector involvement; this could be channelled through the forum, and would be money well spent for informed, representative involvement of the voluntary sector.

CHIs can produce neighbourhood or community constituencies through their broad remits of promoting health, channelling and enabling their communities to give voice to their needs, demands and aspirations. It is therefore crucial that CHIs are included in any voluntary sector forum on health.

Community unit managers should ensure that if they go down this road of accountability in the joint planning process that they stress the importance and advantages of involvement to CHIs and other health related voluntary sector organizations, as many do not wish to get involved with DHAs due to past exploitative experiences. They need to know what they can gain from such involvement. At present access to JCCs is the only route to central decision making available to the voluntary sector.

(iv) Care in the community initiatives

Health authorities are increasingly using the voluntary sector to launch care in the community initiatives. The most common reason given for this is that more flexible responses to peoples' needs can be made to enable them to live 'independently' or 'supported' in the community; it also has the added bonus of being able to attract funds from other sources, e.g. local authority, Joint Finance, the Housing Corporation, Department of Environment, urban programme.

Many DHAs are setting up in partnership with housing associations, local authorities and voluntary sector organizations to establish new voluntary sector initiatives offering accommodation and support packages, e.g. group homes, residential units, independent living schemes. These may or may not have statutory sector staff seconded to them and/or may employ their own staff through the voluntary organization. Some even use volunteers. At best they can offer a real alternative to institutional care and more control for clients, at worst they can represent decentralization to smaller units only, with little loss of medical/professional control over clients' lives. The latter are usually found in those organizations that have little involvement from the voluntary sector, no user involvement and whose priorities are management of resources only.

Other ways that DHAs can support care in the community is by supporting and expanding existing voluntary sector provision, e.g. self-help groups, CHIs, care attendant schemes, respite schemes, volunteer visiting/befriending/counselling schemes. It is important that community unit managers get to know, forge partnerships and work with local voluntary community organizations.

(v) Decentralization and local accountability

The decentralization of general management and community health services provides many opportunities for closer working with the voluntary sector. It also gives workers and managers the chance to get to know their patches better – the population mix, housing, health, local facilities and amenities, and perhaps most importantly the level and type of organized local community action. In the past, managers, planners, and to some extent, fieldworkers in the NHS, largely through ignorance of the voluntary sector, have failed to make any productive links with it. The advent of 'mini' general managers, neighbourhood nursing and other teams, as well as the duty of health authorities to identify community needs and to develop local integrated solutions all mean that the conditions necessary for forging partnerships and joint objectives might have arrived.

Locality planning is providing an opportunity for CHIs and other voluntary organizations to become more involved in and to work closer with community units and community health staff and managers. Exeter CHC, in partnership with Exeter Health Authority, has pioneered locality planning teams consisting of local professionals and lay people to advise locality managers and to be involved in priority setting. There are also health forums throughout the District made up entirely of lay people and community groups. These forums in turn link into some locality planning teams and, indeed, as they have grown in confidence, some are amalgamating with those locality teams (Exeter CHC, 1986). Islington Borough Council in London has 'gone local', with neighbourhood teams of all council services operating from neighbourhood offices, and with input from a neighbourhood committee that has been constituted under their equal opportunities policy to ensure representation of local communities that are traditionally under-represented; these committees also manage a community budget of £2000. Islington HA is decentralizing its community unit to the same boundaries as the borough council and will be siting some of its facilities in the same buildings. A pilot scheme in West Lambeth (Dun, 1987, 1989) advocated the establishment of health forums/alliances based on neighbourhoods (fieldworker levels) and on localities (officer/middle management levels), that could feed into JCCs, JCPTs, CHCs, local authority health sub-committees and District Health Promotion Groups (i.e. at senior officer/management and/or policy-making levels). What these proposals all have in common is that they actively involve local communities, CHIs and voluntary organizations in planning processes, they are inter-sectoral in nature, and hopefully – but especially if they involve the voluntary sector – will keep in mind broad definitions of health and the need for integrated, collective action. Thus, the 'going local' of community unit services can offer a further route to effective partnerships with CHIs. Without input to central policy and senior management decisions, and without the devolution of some power to local forums/planning teams, such as community budgets (as in Islington) or direct involvement in planning that goes beyond consultation, such forums will become talking shops only and participants will lose heart and withdraw.

CHIs and voluntary groups can become more directly involved in their local NHS facilities through user participation groups, local advisory groups, and centre advisory groups (Wilce, 1988) based on health centres, health clinics, community hospitals, community mental health centres.

(vi) Service contracts

Service contracts between District Health Authorities and the voluntary sector provide formalized and structured ways of working together. Whilst they can be viewed as a threat to the autonomy of CHIs they do spell out what each side expects from the other and therefore lessen the ambiguities and misunderstandings that often blight partnerships. They are however becoming a fact of life for many voluntary organizations, and for some can mean the attachment of 'strings' by the funding body through a stipulation of what services should be supplied by the organization.

Community units should employ Voluntary Sector Grants Liaison Officers in the same way that local authorities do, not only to help them to budget, forecast and monitor finances, but also to offer advice on general project management. The NHS, as a funder of CHIs has a responsibility to offer guidance and support to CHIs to ensure that projects are properly managed and financed. Also, many organizations do not have the resources or skills to negotiate in their own favour. CHIs should be advised that outside help is available to them from organizations such as the National Council for Voluntary Organizations and the National Community Health Resource. There should also be a facility in budgets for CHIs training needs to include the management and running of a voluntary organization (if appropriate), and the development of negotiating skills.

FAILURES – AN ANALYSIS OF SOME COMMON PROBLEMS

The following are actual experiences of failure and of demise, and the lessons that those involved learned along the way. Some, but not all, have been recorded.

1. Speke Neighbourhood Health Project was one of those set up by the Foundation of Alternatives, in 1977. The project was chaired by a community physician, and the Speke Neighbourhood Health Group employed a worker and had a membership made up of representatives from the health authority, local authority, CHC, local voluntary sector, DHSS, probation, police and local press. It called for action from the health and local authorities on specfic local health issues. But it never had any official commitment to the project and its aims from the District Health Authority, and in 1983, the reorganization of the DHA provided them with the opportunity 'no longer [to] have formal involvement with the Neighbourhood Council', and it subsequently faded away. It could be said that problems facing this neighbourhood health project stemmed from an attempt to root it in official NHS structures (this was never achieved), rather than its being more 'community' based and growing from local community action. However, three years after its

demise community health action is re-emerging in Speke, centred on a local Women's Health Action Group's call for a health centre and involvement in the planning process (Scott-Samuel, 1989).

2.   A community health worker attached to a health centre and funded through 'soft' funding for two years was held to be too 'political' by the DHA in her work with women and black people. Her funding and post were not taken up by the health authority at the end of the financial period despite written letters of support from other community health workers and local communities. A commitment to project aims and objectives and to continued funding if agreed targets were met would have reduced the vulnerability and ensured the survival of this post.

3.   A community health worker with community development experience in social services departments found that her management was to be transferred to the manager of the health centre to which she was attached. She felt this would cause a conflict of loyalty as her role was to enable users to constructively criticize the centre's running and services. There was also confusion regarding her role which the DHA management saw as essentially public relations, involving local volunteers in the centre, and generally encouraging individuals and groups to use the centre, only; on the other hand the community health worker wished to be accountable to the local advisory group and saw her main task as essentially working with local groups to enable them to identify and articulate their needs. The upshot was that the CHW resigned and her post was not continued – despite support from the local advisory group. The lessons here could be ones of confusion over lines of responsibility and management, lack of clarity in the job description, and differences in approach and aims. An NHS management structure for NHS employed community health workers could help to avoid such confusion.

4.   A short-term pilot project with 'soft' funding was set up by a DHA planning department to look at different approaches to the planning and delivery of primary and community health services. The grading of the post meant that the worker had insufficient status to make recommendations and effect change within the DHA. A combination of NHS reorganization, frequent change of management, lack of DHA commitment to the principles of the project,

together with a too generalized job description left the worker with lack of direction, lack of belonging to either the NHS or the voluntary sector; this in turn led to feelings of being isolated, marginalized and essentially powerless. Her well researched reports and recommendations were largely ignored and the project failed to make much impact locally. A commitment by the project's aims and to follow up research findings would have avoided the unnecessary waste of work and resources.

The more successful CHIs have grown out of local community action and as such are rooted in a response to community needs, such as the Stockwell Health Project that grew from local activity around a proposed health centre; Glyndon Health Rights Project from a local CHC based community health survey; Tower Hamlets Health Project from a local health enquiry. Those that fail have often been imposed on communities. Successful CHIs also have clear aims and objectives that local communities 'own' and have a vested interest in. These community-based CHIs usually only disappear through lack of funding or if they have come to a natural end – they are rarely open to sabotage. Such projects are organic in nature and exist whether funded or not, wherever need is great enough for people to feel impelled to organize in order to effect local action. What is new is the recognition of a movement wth a growing identity, namely the Community Health Movement. The potential of this movement is the sharing of experiences, mutual support, growing self-confidence and the solidarity necessary to challenge medical institutions in order for local communities, women, black people, and other discriminated against groups to reclaim their health. This is a legitimate role for CHIs.

The NHS role in CHIs could arguably be more critically analysed. The failure of the NHS and the CHM at present to clarify this is producing NHS sponsored posts and projects that have no clear idea of where they are coming from or where they are going. The lack of community development strategies and clearly stated policies or job descriptions is leaving many newly created NHS based CHWs outside of NHS and voluntary sector structures. Instead of setting up these posts and projects as quasi-voluntary sector ones, DHAs need to be sure whether they should be rooted in the NHS or the voluntary sector and choose one or the other. If voluntary sector-based, workers must be accountable to local management committees who manage the funding, staffing, contract(s) of employment, policies and targets, within aims and objectives agreed with funding bodies (e.g. DHA) and subject to appropriate evaluation, that is 'arms-length' funding and control that ensure their autonomy. If NHS-based, CHIs and CHWs should be properly managed by an appropriate manager. Within a DHA, commitment to a community development approach and statements of intent, together with an overall community development strategy and relevant structures, are essential if the worker is to be productive.

The relationship between health authorities and the voluntary sector will necessitate negotiation. One side will require certain services, functions and ratification of policies, whilst the other will be seeking funding and professional support, as well as recognition. What is needed is clarity of purpose on both sides. Each will need to establish, at each encounter, who is setting the agenda and what are the aims and objectives of each meeting, working party, steering group, and what each side wants from such a partnership, together with an openness as to what they have to contribute. A certain amount of candour is necessary, particularly regarding the limitations and restrictions imposed on participants, for example, how much funding, if any, is available, whether there is official policy and commitment to support partnership proposals, and what structures and pathways exist to enable action. This will all go some way towards avoiding the exploitation that can be felt when information is withheld; it will also foster confidence and build trust. The voluntary sector could, by adopting legitimate lobbying and campaigning activities denied to health authority professionals, provide routes for frustrated health authority staff seeking to change policy. Similarly health authority participants could foster understanding of voluntary sector activity inside the health authority, as well as championing jointly agreed goals and funding for voluntary sector activity.

The NHS and voluntary sector, even though they might have similar goals, have different cultures. Their experiences are likely to be ones of competing for limited resources and of conflict. However, with clarity of expectations, that is, what each side hopes to achieve from each encounter, together with the sharing and pooling of ideas, experiences and resources, joint goals can be identified and achieved. Achievements, however small, can cement relationships and engender mutual respect. These can be built upon. Failures, if examined with similar candour, can yield many lessons that aid partnership construction.

A VISION FOR THE FUTURE

This final section will outline two ways in which work with and through the CHM by DHAs might be enhanced. While structures and good management are necessary, good processes including honesty, commitment and a genuine desire to work with the community are indispensible.

Towards a model for voluntary sector based, NHS funded CHIs

Funding should be long term where possible and either of an 'arms-length' type or made via contractual arrangements for services. A useful model or starting point could be developed from proposals suggested by NAHA/NCVO (NAHA, 1988). These suggest that every health authority should develop a policy for promoting closer links with the voluntary sector that has the full commitment from the health authority, together with a strong lead 'from the top'. The appointment of designated officers with the responsibility for developing links and partnerships with the voluntary sector is proposed; together with a policy towards the voluntary sector that includes: a general statement of intent; the identification of groups and procedures through which consultation and planning will take place; and specific policies relating to grants and grants procedures, the use and loan of premises and equipment. Health authorities might also create 'Voluntary Sector Grants Liaison Officer' posts to aid the distribution and monitoring of grants. A model of the sort of processes that might and voluntary sector and CHI in district planning is presented as Figure 5.1.

Towards a model for NHS based community development and CHIs

District Health Authorities should adopt the principles of WHO Health For All proposals for a community development approach. A district-wide Community Development Officer post could be created at senior level in order to provide coherent management

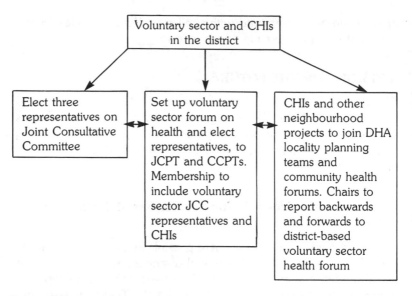

Figure 5.1 Schematic diagram of possible voluntary sector routes to DHA planning process

and support to community health workers and NHS initiated CHIs. Decentralized community units could employ a CHW for each locality and/or neighbourhood whose job would be to set up and service interagency locality planning teams and to support and, where necessary, initiate and aid the seeking of funding for community and voluntary sector based CHIs. Other CHW posts could be set up attached to a local health facility, such as a health centre or community care centre with the task of serving the centre catchment area, to initiate a user group or local advisory group, and community development based on the health facility. A main role of CHWs wll be to aid the autonomy and self-help elements of CHIs whilst offering themselves as resources. There must be a written commitment by DHAs and community units actively to involve local communities. CHWs would be managed by the Senior Community Development Officer and would have parity as far as job descriptions and salaries are concerned. Grants Liaison Officers would be available to aid CHIs to obtain and monitor funding as well as to plan and budget finances. Community unit staff will need to have job descriptions and training to include skills necessary for group work, community development and working with the voluntary sector. At all levels the statement of DHA commitment to community development and participation will impact on working practices and attitudes. Structures are important. They minimize confusion and ambiguity; people know where they stand and instead of imposing strictures, they foster strength and facilitate the taking of initiatives. Similar models are to be found in local authorities. These have a long history of partnership with the voluntary sector, of community development, and of the debates around 'patch' working methods. Figure 5.2 suggests a possible community development management structure for a District Health Authority.

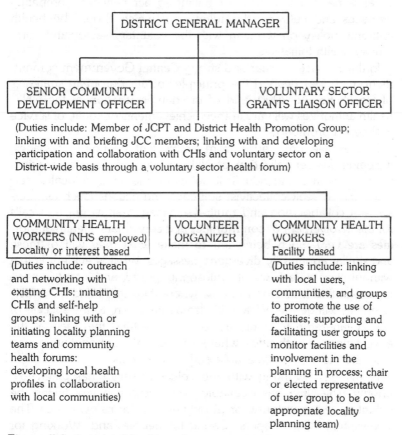

Figure 5.2 Suggested health authority community development structure

CONCLUSION

Clearly the entrepreneurial community unit general manager has much to gain from the voluntary sector. There is sufficient benefit to be gained from the formation of such partnerships for the pragmatist to know it makes sense, and for the idealist to know that it is desirable. Just as general management can provide a counterbalance to doctors, so can CHIs benefit the NHS. This is particularly pertinent at a time when criticism is being levelled at the NHS that the scales have been tipped in its and in the doctors' favour for too long and that reform and a focus on consumers is overdue. What is needed is a kind of balancing act between competing demands and cultures, the fulcrum of which should be health authority policy on working with the voluntary sector and community health initiatives.

In the absence of clear and strong Central Government commitment, that goes beyond the principles of the European strategies of Health For All 2000, and of the democratization of the NHS, health authorities will vary in their achievements of equity of service and health promotion.

Further dilemmas arise from ambivalent centralist messages, including the centralization of NHS policy and decision making, the promotion of individualistic solutions, the drive to localize services and to seek collectivist solutions and actions (such as intersectoral collaboration and multi-disciplinary teamwork), and calls for the involvement of communities and consumers. Health authorities are very much being left to make what they will of these and similar apparently divergent messages. What is evident is that without clear statements of philosophy, policy, and intent, participants will find it difficult to know where they stand and misunderstandings will be rife. What will also be necessary to the success of any collaboraton is clarity as to who is setting the agenda, the expectations of both sides, what is on the table for negotiation, and what are the jointly achievable and agreed goals.

In the past, working with the voluntary sector has taken low priority. The NHS has justifiably been accused of not taking the voluntary sector seriously or of only using it for its own ends. The government White Papers 'Caring for people' and 'Working for patients' both see the voluntary sector as playing a major role in the provision of health and social care. Serious approaches will not only need commitment but wll also demand time. Is this going to be feasible for a time-limited, product-orientated manager? Are managers able to make such commitments to communities and voluntary organizations? It is probably too early to tell.

A major function of the community unit is to provide services, and that of the community health movement is to promote health. Solutions sought in the absence of the voluntary sector and CHIs are likely only to address those of service delivery and management. Without the involvement of CHIs and other forms of lay representation there is little to indicate that general management, localization and streamlined services will do much to advance health. They might improve the lot of health professionals, management and Department of Health budgets. They might even improve access for some to services. However, they are unlikely to make much difference to district or national health on their own. In fact the NHS alone cannot achieve the advancement of health of local populations, as this relies on too many societal and environmental factors that are outside of NHS control.

Clearly the advancement of health requires a will to work with the voluntary sector, and for community units to work with their health education/promotion departments, with local GPs and other family practioner committee services, with the Community Health Council, the local authority social services, housing, environmental health and committees on health, with hospital-based services and with residential units. In short it requires broader definitions of health and broader-based strategies and solutions.

There needs to be a change in the way the NHS and those employed by it work, and in how decisions are made. Health authorities and community units working with the voluntary sector is focal to such change.

6

Working with local authorities

Glenn Warren and Jenny Harrow

The rationale for joint working between health authorities, providing 'health care', and local authorities providing 'social services' and 'housing', is increasingly consumerist. Health and health-related needs do not respect organizationally defined boundaries. Service 'clients', 'patients' or, the more neutral term, 'users', face confusion in confronting inter-organizational boundaries, and, when (rarely) asked, overwhelmingly opt for the identification of 'key workers' to guide them through the responsibility maze, if not to ensure improved service quality (Ferlie, Pahl and Quine, 1987) 'Overlap' is a familiar occurrence; for example, much of the community support provided by health authority auxiliary nursing staff may also be provided by social services departments' domiciliary care staff, such as bathing and night sitting services. 'Who does what' often depends upon with which agency the individual's contact, or referral, was first made, a situation providing for duplication in some circumstances, patchy or non-existent services in others, and one in which users are ill-served, until co-ordination takes some hold.

This recognition, perhaps tardy, that 'the customer knows best', occurs at a time when health care costs are under scrutiny. Is there a country in the Western hemisphere which can afford the quality of health care which professionals have the knowledge and the skills to provide? The 1980s have been a period of little or no growth in the UK's health service. This has produced continual reappraisal of the manner in which health care resources are used, with increasing emphasis on the need to integrate services provided by health authorities and complementary services supported, in particular, by local authorities.

This chapter illustrates these themes by considering the nature of 'joint working' and the managerial skills it demands; reviewing the experiences and results of joint working from a variety of practitioner and academic perspectives; examining the opportunities for opening up joint working to public participation through reference to North Staffordshire Health Authority's Neighbourhood Forum work; and finally by discussing the likelihood of increasing authoritative strategies on the part of Central Government to ensure inter-organizational collaboration.

JOINT WORKING AND ITS MANAGERIAL DEMANDS

As consumers 'go public' over the loose fit of statutory services – the patient discharged inappropriately to a cold, empty home during a weekend, against the background of measuring acute hospitals' performance by their bed occupancy rates – the services which are held to 'need integration' are increasingly under pressure, as workloads are stretched in response to demographic change. Joint planning mechanisms for health and social services have existed in the UK since the mid-70s, with the impressively titled Joint Care Planning Teams seen in the majority of health districts as ways of distributing Joint Finance, but with little attempt to engage in joint strategic planning. Joint Finance, introduced in 1977 'as a way of using health service money to oil the wheels of joint planning and enable new community based services to be developed' (Harding, 1986), was recognized in a 1985 DHSS working party report on joint planning as 'often used in a piecemeal way, often unrelated to an overall plan of joint finance development' (DHSS, 1985).

It seems likely that notions of joint funding as providing a 'quick capital fix' in certain situations are strong; although Joint Finance represents only approximately 1% of health service budgets and 3% of social services budgets. Even for those who comprehend the range of 'Joint Planning' and 'Joint Finance' acronyms, it is of little comfort that at both policy planning and policy delivery levels a chronic lack of linkage between health and social services is a European-wide feature. WHO's Regional Office for Europe published a study of health and welfare co-ordination in Austria, Poland, Sweden and Italy, identifying three key reasons for concern with service linkage (Kohn, 1977). These were: service fragmentation, the growing needs of particular client groups and demands for agency accountability regarding service efficiency and effectiveness. All three aspects are central, ten years on, to the debates on the reality or paucity of 'Community Care' in Britain, and to the most recent Griffiths Report on that area. Any review of collaboration between health authorities and local authorities must also recognize the stake in that work held by the service users and by local voluntary organizations, the latter defined by Harding as 'independent non profit making citizen organisations' (Harding, 1986). As Harding demonstrates, the very range of voluntary sector activity means that its potential contribution to collaborative work will necessarily be complex. The issue of the voluntary sector health contribution is examined more fully in Chapter 5.

The competing perspectives surrounding collaboration require a structure to ensure understanding of the stresses imposed upon those involved in collaborative work; Kohn's three areas are useful in this respect. As this chapter demonstrates, the literature suggests a fragmented development of collaborative projects, dependent upon the enthusiasm of the few. Where the literature shows a concentration on policy agreement, it may also ignore real disharmony among field staff. A sense of ownership of collaborative work amongst planners, managers and members will be as nothing if health authority field staff know 'the social services' only as the people who decline referrals, and vice versa. The extent to which the attempts at collaboration fully address the areas highlighted by Kohn must be recognized as limited.

Joint working can be seen as the practical expression of the recognition that social health-related problems do not come in neat organizationally-based packages. As a term it may be preferable to the more formal 'collaboration', with overtones for some generations, of activities motivated by self-interest and self-preservation. This connotation may in fact have a value: some experience of joint working may be rooted in organizations seeking to survive. Where local authorities are, for example, becoming more wary of taking on Joint Finance based commitments, as the resource provision eventually falls to them after the initial health service funded 'cushion', this is likely to be influenced by their other resource strategies, and not by any sudden rejection of the joint working 'principle'. As Hudson argues convincingly, if depressingly, 'it may be more realistic to assume that inter-organisational collaboration in social welfare has no qualities of spontaneous growth or self perpetuation' (Hudson, 1987).

Any review of opportunities gained and problems encountered in joint health authority-local authority work must therefore be cautious of sermonizing. Altruistic behaviour by key decision makers and professionals 'required' to collaborate, whilst not being ruled out, is not a secure basis for policy development. Joint working needs to be 'managed' like any other health service initiative. It is possible that the skills needed for this are as much those of an earlier generation of 'administrators', functioning in 'consensus management' contexts, as they are of the current 'general managers', with clearer lines of responsibility in relation to clinicians and a more aggressive intervention style. This is likely to be the case, given that if a health authority is strongly committed to joint local authority working, it is likely to lose some of its fully independent base for action and will have to invest energy, over time, in building up inter-organizational contacts before results become apparent. With general managers on fixed contracts, the variety of means by which joint working is 'sold' to health authority members is an issue for investigation in its own right.

OVERVIEW OF EXPERIENCES OF JOINT WORKING

McKeganey and Hunter describe how when any reference occurs to the service needs of the priority care grops – the elderly, the mentally handicapped, the mentally ill – 'improved service co-ordination is invoked almost reflexively' (McKeganey and Hunter, 1986). This increases the likelihood that the gap between joint working intention and joint working delivery may be considerable, but this can be gauged only in part by a review of the progress reported to date in the joint working initiatives so far occurring. Hudson's view that British work on analysing social welfare collaboration has been unduly empirical draws attention to the problems of measuring its impact and effectiveness (Hudson, 1987).

The empirical tradition has perhaps also helped to ensure that joint working between health and local authorities is not headline grabbing. Scunthorpe DHA's experiences of 'joint planning' have been characterized as 'unremarkable but productive', an honest perspective only attractive to the already 'converted' (Nightingale, 1988). The innate modesty in this analysis may disguise the extent to which Nightingale's account of joint planning processes experienced by health, local authorities and voluntary organizations in

Scunthorpe has value, if only because, ironically, it is most open about the degree of 'despondency' experienced by the would-be joint planners. Key areas of concern included membership of the planning group, the alternative accountabilities of the participants, and the existing managerial and structural frameworks within which participants had to work.

After describing 'near collapse', followed by the successful creation of a Mental Health Action Group, Nightingale pinpoints 'the lessons' for others. As his account stresses, the 'unremarkability' of these ideas may mean that their innate value is minimized and their impact lost. Ideas such as 'having a concrete purpose', and a tangible task to work on, 'achieving trust and openness among members', and meeting in 'active informal venues' draw attention to at least two major issues associated with any such joint action. The first is the extent to which these critical commonplaces will or will not attract younger key professionals in either health or local authority service, to the notion that effort greater than that required by statute will 'pay off'. In a period when a career orientation is both expected, and associated with both dramatic and certainly non-incremental activity, an extensive commitment in career terms to joint working initiatives may be – or seem to be – a luxury. What role models for rapid career progression are available for delivering 'slow and steady' joint working, as opposed to simply 'surviving' the known rigours of the joint planning machinery? The second issue is the wider and continuing one of querying the portability of this experience, particularly since the catalyst for eventual 'results' was participant depression and the group's experience of *impasse* and near-collapse. Do wise participants therefore bring their joint planning machinery close to breaking point to 'shake' members into recognition of the losses which would then accrue? Logically, this may be a risk worth taking in some instances; which type of participant should engineer it is an uncertain question.

The critic will have noticed that the above example refers to 'joint planning' rather than 'joint working', and may have assumed that the former is the process which must precede the latter. At the risk of semantic nicety, it is possible to view the two terms as interchangeable. The 'Scunthorpe experience', in Nightingale's terms, provides an example of how 'lubrication' of joint planning processes might occur. One 'lesson' which seems implicit in the account cited above is the extent to which once minor targets were met, more major targets appeared feasible. This finds an important echo in Bryson's recent argument that public service – and voluntary sector – managers should aim for 'small wins' in their strategic planning as part of an overall and eventual 'big win' plan (Bryson, 1988). How many potential joint working participants in any event perceive joint working as representing 'small wins' (when users may regard it, in effect, as 'big wins') is a matter for conjecture.

That joint planning teams must be seen to 'win' – whether on the large or the small scale – when choosing schemes for joint working is stressed by Gale, Garton and Webster (1988) in their practical review and critique of the joint planning process, as seen from the perspective of Cambridgeshire County Council, which inter-relates with four Health Districts and six District Councils. Accepting the continuing uncertainty as to which initiatives might be adopted, because of the differing ways in which participating agencies operate, they emphasize the importance of fully briefing joint planning team members on, for example, criteria which each agency would use to judge a scheme, and guidance on how a scheme should be presented. They note:

> In Cambridgeshire guidelines are issued annually to all joint planning teams, covering timetable, resource availability and selection criteria. They are also given regular updates on the current status of the Health Authorities' and County Council's plans. Housing representatives on the teams are also expected to brief other members.

Their paragraph heading, 'picking the winners', remains, however, a reminder of the extent to which joint planning and working may be seen by some would-be practitioners and collaborators as a gamble, in time, money and effort. The apparent linkage between increases in capital investment and independent reviews from bodies such as the Hospital Advisory Service is a reminder of how 'progress' is seen to many to be related to the provision of buildings and not to the quality of relationships bult up over time between various agency representatives.

Where health authorities are seen as more likely to be 'leading' the joint working processes, because of their resource base, as compared with other potential 'workers' (if not their more innovative managers), this has occasioned some criticism. In teamwork terms, dominant 'leadership' by one group may mean 'lack of ownership' of ideas, activities and possible solutions by the other groups, with perhaps correspondingly less commitment to the decisions and less effort to maintain momentum for change. The notion of 'ownership' is well understood in group settings. 'Identification with' an approach or proposal has a similar meaning. It is difficult to identify research which shows what this lack of 'ownership' amounts to in joint working operations and precisely how it manifests itself, and whether its results are all deleterious.

If any one group has a greater ownership element of plans and actions, this may cause imbalance in the notion of 'teams', encouraging more effort to be placed to ensure intra-organization parity rather than joint working. This will occur only if health authorities take an 'ownership' line. In an extensively documented example of interagency collaboration where the lead agency has been local authority social services departments – the All-Wales Strategy for Services for Mentally Handicapped People – health authority personnel have in some settings worked under what appears an imposed 'consensus', by virtue of the presence of the Director of Social Services as chair of the relevant Planning and Development Group (McGrath, 1988). By implication here, health authority staff may have found collaboration more complex if only because they will represent a number of health perspectives from within their authority, whereas an apparent unity of ideas may come from the social services department.

For those despairing of joint working in England having some central thrust and support (other than, perhaps, the reduction of long-stay hospital provision), the AWS appears to provide an appealing model. Centralization of responsibility for both health and social services lies within the Welsh Office, and, as Hunter and Wistow (1987) document fully, Treasury funding mechanisms for block grant funding for Wales enable the Welsh Office to shift around its funds to emphasize its favoured policies. Begun in 1983, it has been backed by central (i.e. Welsh Office) funding for innovative projects, aiming to 'recast' services for mentally handicaped people upon principles of 'normalization', with funding for 1988–89 running at £13m (Welsh Office, 1983). The argument that 'real' joint working is more likely to occur once a focus has been taken for a particular client group is well illustrated by this policy; some commentators regard its shifting responsibility towards local authorities and emphasize inter-service co-ordination as, in effect, a 'tryout' of the Griffiths proposals for community care services (Hudson, 1988).

The scale of the AWS work, and the leverage which the centrally-backed policy has had on those statutory agencies is impressive, with the existing **structures** for joint working but no particular commitment to making those structures produce operational plans. However, a review of the work undertaken at the micro as opposed to macro level of the All-Wales Strategy in operation produces evidence of problems with joint working that are all too familiar. McGrath (1988) reported on part of a DHSS research programme evaluating one of the two 'Vanguard' areas for the AWS (one in South Wales, one in Gwynedd). She focused on the activities of the 'P and D' group, the Planning and Development Group, responsible for planning comprehensive services for mentally handicapped people in particular districts, and the release of Welsh Office funds depending on its approval of these plans. Inter-agency differences in managerial styles and devolutionary practices created problems, even when 'apparent consensus' at the group meetings concealed these. For example, whilst health authority staff sought greater 'say' over budgets for local managers, budgetary arrange-ments within the county council meant that this was neither feasible nor appropriate for their local managers. Ominously, she noted that 'Many of the proposals in the plans have have not yet been developed sufficiently for inter-organisational difficulties to arise' (McGrath, 1988, p. 56).

When switching to review the operational level of the AWS, the 'Service Delivery group', comprising 11 health authority and eight local authority officers, McGrath notes a similar picture, whilst reporting a harsher verdict from participants on its working: 'a disaster', 'a shambles' (McGrath, 1988, p. 59).

The symbolic importance of apparently simple issues, difficult to resolve, is highlighted. For example, mail is opened centrally, logged and then distributed within social services departments, an unacceptable practice for health service managers. With elected members in Gwynedd making all social services appointments, the social services department was unable to offer the health authority involvement in joint appointments of staff. McGrath reports firmly the degree of learning from the 'health' side of the constraints facing local authorities, but this learning is itself frustrating, as the

limits which these constraints impose on collaboration are identified.

With a framework for collaboration in place, McGrath identifies
two key elements which now required:

1. Commitment to make collaboration work, the willingness to
   implement decisions; and
2. The ability to implement decisions.

Commitment is seen in part as a function of staff involvement in
planning processes; and restructuring changes for the Gwynedd
collaboration proposed in 1988 are examined, not only within
social services but also in the health authority where 'reorganisation
currently taking place . . . will leave one person responsible for
mentally handicapped services' (McGrath, 1988, p. 65). Against this
background of detailed uncertainty is the awareness that the Welsh
Office backing has helped induce efforts to 'jointly plan' where
these were previously minimal, so ensuring a widening of service
perspective which in medium and longer terms will be likely to
'repay'.

At the same time, the extent to which the AWS does **not** provide
a complete 'success story' is useful inasmuch as it indicates that
'lack of funding' is not the sole and major barrier to change. The
problems of **intra**-organizational relations, in both the health
authority and the local authority, were highlighted (for example,
with the latter, the very limited involvement of the education department); but how such problems should be best handled remains
open to question. Whether any efforts to work jointly should be
shelved until improved intra-organizational understanding on policy
stances be obtained, or whether joint working should proceed, in
the full knowledge that intra-organizational disagreement provides
plenty of internal policy progress tripwires is presumably always a
matter for local judgement. It is also perhaps important to note that
in the reviews chosen above, the education department's 'voice'
and perspective on its stand was not made explicit, so that its
unwilling involvement as such cannot be inferred.

That social services departments should always be the 'lead
agency' from **within** the local authority seems appropriate, because
of those departments' multiclient and multidisciplinary concerns;
but this may not necessarily be so; and in a number of instances
education departments may be the more appropriate 'internal lead'

department. Examples of health authority/education authority joint working should support this, for example the experiments in Maidstone and Medway Health Districts taking mobile health clinic services to Traveller sites, in collaboration with Kent Education Committee (Pahl and Vaile, 1988).

McGrath's conclusion – that if the complex interagency co-ordination problems in AWS are to be resolved, 'considerable managerial skills will be required' – begs the question as to which groupings of skills these are and among which range of managers they need to be located. Implicit in some of the discussion about the internal workings of AWS is the suggestion that 'joint working' needs to start **within** the existing collaborating authorities as a prior condition to successful joint working with **external** bodies. This is perhaps as much a matter of strongly held differing professional perspectives on service priorities as any low commitment to joint working.

This is a view echoed by Ferlie, Pahl and Quine in their arguments for 'key workers' for mentally handicapped people, and for 'outward looking' joint work, not limited by organizational boundaries, and for example 'accepting referrals from any one' (Ferlie, Pahl and Quine, 1987). They write: 'It is not our intention to decry the idea of joint planning and joint working, nor to suggest that this way of organizing services should be abandoned. However at present large numbers of expensive professionals are spending a considerable amount of time in the many interdisciplinary meetings which joint working implies. Our concern is that their time should be spent as effectively as possible.'

Setting aside the question of 'how many' of the 'expensive professionals' are really so involved – and whether all would class themselves as 'expensive' – such a stance would seem to suggest that the managerial skills needed in such settings are those which can set aside or over-ride interprofessional disharmony; or are they perhaps those associated with willingness to accept a degree of deprofessionalization? For some commentators, the barriers which justify professionals' existence and power are at the heart of joint working failures. Green (1986), for example, quotes extensively from other writers to support this viewpoint, concluding that 'Joint Finance and schemes like it will continue to enjoy only limited success' without reform to eliminate the legal privileges on which professional power rests.

Certainly the moment at which joint working is referred to, whether informally or in formal documentation as a 'partnership', a term both growing in use and reflecting the practicalities of the degree of 'input' given by informal 'carers', some tenets of professional behaviour are open to challenge. Sensitivity to the need for professionals in both health and social services spheres to explain why they feel a certain course of action may be appropriate may, for example, be in short supply. It is also possible that some 'real' joint working has foundered on what might be called 'managerial incompetence', from among the best of motives, whether among health service or social service personnel, in deference to known professional susceptibilities – the managerial skills of calming down debate, 'seeing the other's point of view', smoothing over disagreements, but in so doing ensuring that any number of key issues are not debated fully, and a proper 'joint' perspective never fully reached. For some harassed and over-stretched managers in both health and social services, a definition of 'successful' joint working might well be where no major challenges are ever issued to either 'side', and the respective 'boats' are not 'rocked'.

JOINT WORKING AND PUBLIC PARTICIPATION

Given that a fundamental rationale for joint working is the improvement – qualitatively and then perhaps quantitatively – of service from the user or consumer perspective, 'users' or 'consumers' as an interested 'group' represent in practice another important element in the local authority/health authority working relationship. That some statutory agency professionals feel uneasy when working with, as opposed to working 'for', their service users may be for some sufficient argument for ensuring that the consumer perspective is well heard in any joint working system. No-one ever said that joint working was supposed to be easy! Models of joint working may be seen to approach consumerist involvement from a variety of directions: they may take it 'as read', since they can expect to be lobbied by relevant groups; they may seek to incorporate it through offering membership of joint planning groups to representatives of formal bodies, such as local branches of national voluntary organizations; or they may aim to establish consumer/user participation from across a wide spectrum at the 'pre-planning' stage, so that consumer views are central to the subsequent planning and work, rather than tailored to fit professionals' thinking as a valuable adjunct.

The last-named approach will be seen as the most valuable and justifiable for increasing the validity of policies chosen and implemented. Nevertheless, in practice, the involvement of service consumers (whether as 'patients', 'clients' or as families/friends) in joint working adds to the complexity of the process. It may add to the professional's constant fear – 'heightened expectations' – and may limit the degree of frank exchange between professionals. Even where user participation has been a central element in a joint working arena, rather than grafted on subsequently, its impact is not guaranteed and its popularity may be open to question. The issue of the personal energy required for a continuing commitment to involvement in joint planning, by service consumers should not be under-estimated.

Humphreys' review of the development of parental participation in the All-Wales Strategy, where the planning mode had been designed to be one of partnership, shows the variety of parental response (Humphreys, 1987). Even in the AWS' Vanguard districts, participation levels by parents only reached between 30–40%, and were followed by 'gradual disengagement of parents from the planning process'. As with joint working, voices raised against participative activity are negligible, but the value of embarking on participation based exercises may always be open to question. In the case of the AWS, Humphreys points to a further central dilemma – that it is a policy initiative seeking to invigorate democracy at the local level whilst seeking also to ensure the effective implementation of a centralist policy. The same might be said to be the case for local efforts to involve consumers in the decisions about patterns of community care for their localities.

For some practitioners, the joint planning/joint working 'maze' can only be made more complex by the injection of consumer opinion. In practice this may actually delay joint activities from 'taking off', by revealing all too clearly the fundamental differences between professionals within services, professionals in alternative or parallel services and professionals and clients/users/patients. No participative activity is free of this risk, and whilst some destabilization and challenging of traditional relationships may be a necessary precursor for 'true' joint planning, it may be the brave managers who are willing to sit out the short-term disagreements which may surface, in order to gain the higher moral ground of full involvement of the users for whom the service is intentionally provided.

The logic of this would seem to be that the value of a participative user 'base' for joint working needs to be stated and provided for at the beginning of a joint working relationship. This approach would seem to be a good base from which to 'pick the winners' for joint working, emphasized above; not only should the extent of shortfalls in service be seen, but both realistic and popular proposals made. An extensive development on these lines, with the establishment of Neighbourhood Health Forums, has taken place in North Staffordshire Health Authority, under the aegis of the Authority's Community Services Unit. This followed the example from Exeter Health Authority, with its work on what has become known as Locality Planning, although with the former, the relevant local authorities were not involved from the beginning of the project (King, 1986; Exeter and District Community Health Council, 1986).

The Neighbourhood Forum concept, as operating in North Staffordshire since Spring 1988, is designed to enable the public identification of the major issues relating to health needs in community settings. By definition these are not amenable to the existing organizational boundaries and rules of service provision, **prior** to 'top-down' decisions being taken on what a particular locale 'needs'. The degree of consistency thus far demonstrated from the four currently operating, two based in rural market towns and two in the Potteries towns of Stoke on Trent and Newcastle Under Lyme, indicates the value of this. The needs of elderly people and the availability of information on services have been identified in all of these as key areas for work.

Any public airing of such issues may generate additional work for already hard-pressed staff in their own existing specialist areas. It may also gloss over the administrative strains of joint planning or working proposals (the cry, once again of the 'expensive professionals'). In North Staffordshire HA therefore, internal managerial devolution within the Community Unit was seen as an important precursor to the establishment of any new structure designed to facilitate more public involvement and, potentially, more criticism. In effect, the health authority's own staff needed to be 'sold' ideas stressing the value of **their** participation in areas of internal authority decision making. The value of restructuring internal managerial prior to any notions of 'going public' must be stressed. Thus internal structural change within the Authority's Community Services took place, reflecting and responding to staff opinions, over a period of four months, as an important *a priori* condition before the establishment of any external forum.

The success of this 'selling exercise' to staff by the Community Unit General Manager has been reviewed by Warren (1987). Initial staff hesitancy would seem to have been replaced by increasing internal support. Issues raised in the Neighbourhood Forums receive a stronger response than under the previously centralized machinery. Once a degree of internal devolution had been established, the Health Authority contracted the University of Keele Department of Geography to identify 'natural' neighbourhood boundaries; they identified 35, varying in population size from 8000 to 20 000. In the four now in operation, local (health) managers were invited to contact a range of individuals living or working in the area to commence the forum's work. This degree of 'selective participation', whilst open to criticism, and certainly not completely representative, ensured the range of interest in the forums' work. The meetings had loose agendas and allowed the exchange of ideas on the major issues on health affecting the neighbourhood.

The creation of Neighbourhood Health Forums on their own no more guarantees 'proper' choices for joint working, or ensuring that existing resources are deployed with most effect, notably when duplication and overlap may occur, than did the Joint Planning and Funding machinery when set up in 1976. Any structures designed to facilitate joint strategic planning and working will only be as effective as the agencies supporting them wish them to be, and as operating structures **below** them allow them to be. They do not represent pre-requisites for joint working, but an important managerial acknowledgement that the needs and demands of would-be and actual service users, articulated in 'local' contexts, provide critical insights into services duplication, overlap or absence, pointing to joint working directions that may well be 'winners'.

It would be wrong to suggest that the forums are, as yet, identifying the aspects which residents feel are important. In the first instance, their major impact has been the coming together of those who work in the neighbourhoods, and their joint identification of health needs, whether from voluntary, local authority or individual perspectives. Thus, the forum concept gives legitimacy to the consumer viewpoint in settings other than those which are heavily 'committee based'. This is the experience in much joint planning work, where 'consumer representatives' may be heavily outnumbered by the professionals. The forums' activities so far to lie with forum members, chaired by those other than health service staff, albeit recognizable 'community leaders' or spokesmen – local councillors, a senior school headmaster, and so on. At the same time, locality managers inviting local people to initial forum meetings were not always well received. This indicates the extent to which a degree of managerial risk always accompanies 'open invitations' to such public involvement, if only in terms of sustaining hard-pressed managers' morale, and commitment to getting closer to their customers.

The forums certainly give opportunities for particular 'axe grinding'. Disgruntled health users or workers, whether in health or other public services, may attempt to displace its work and use it as a vehicle for generally 'pressurizing' the health authority, or, indirectly, the local social services and housing authorities. In deliberately setting out to reflect a 'neighbourhood' view this system may on occasion fragment opinion and set neighbourhoods against each other. However legitimate the decisions on 'neighbourhood' size and designation, not all will identify with the neighbourhoods 'given' and give rise to further difficulty. In North Staffordshire, for example, the Association of Moorlands Parish Councils, whilst welcoming the concept, sees the neighbourhoods as set out as too large. Just as Joint Planning machinery has been criticized for becoming moribund or operating in perfunctory fashion, so the Neighbourhood Forum concept has within it the opportunity for 'discussions about discussions' rather than promoting specific activities. They may be useful 'sounding boards' but little more.

The issue of the cost of forum establishment remains problematic. Initial spending has been minimal, with approximately £3000 spent on the University of Keele's work, but with the time of health service managers in forum establishment varying. When based on those managers' direct contacts, it represents roughly a week of their time, spread over a month; other managers have taken less time by making greater use of the telephone and contact by letter in establishing the initial groundwork. Interestingly, thus far there seems to be little difference in the forums' 'success' in terms of initial start-up approaches used. Hall hire, refreshment costs, borne by the health authority, are again small. As all the forums have spawned working groups, to focus on particular service areas, there are likely to be increasing costs in supporting the forums with senior managers' time once they are fully 'up and running'.

The newness of the approach in North Staffordshire, where only a handful of forums are in operation, means that the stage of 'disappointment' has perhaps yet to be reached. Local councillors' involvement has been so far been enthusiastic, and it is possible to see greater involvement with local authorities developing if only because of the support for the forums by local voluntary organizations. For the forums to retain their initial impetus and membership involvement, there must be not only airing of problems but action and practical response to the problems raised. Without this it would be possible for their sessions simply to mirror the experiences of all sorts of joint planning/working structures, reflecting good will and little more. Gale, Garton and Webster's (1988) practical and witty guide for the staff member, only belatedly told that they are 'representing the department' on the joint planning team for 'good things', raises questions that might equally apply to forum work:

- Where am I?
- Who are all these people?
- What is the purpose of the group?
- What contribution can I make?
- Who is going to take any notice of the group?

Thus far, neighbourhood involvement or locality planning for joint working generally receives a welcome because its introduction may be seen to signal a degree of seriousness in the joint working field. The 'bottom-up' rather than 'top-down' policy making approach will more accurately reflect users' needs rather than the limited compromises and 'nods' which practitioners, left to themselves, might devise. Whilst inexpensive in the short run, its costs may increase if and when senior managers and health care practitioners respond to forum requests and demands. It has a clear facility for focusing on particularly key needs in communities. Whether its extensive use as a joint working base may also in time further lessen the efforts for the 'less popular' users or clients is a matter for conjecture. The DHSS Working Party report on Disturbed Adolescents (1988) notes the extent to which this user group was already excluded from many existing joint planning systems, whilst particularly commending the locality planning work in Exeter, and proposed work in Dudley:

> Visiting teams were unable to detect plans for disturbed young people that in any way compared with those that had been developed . . . e.g. for adult mental health, for old people.

It is this report which also explicitly notes with regret in relation to planning the discovery of 'so few examples of the positive involvement of Community Health Councils in planning . . . [Some visits revealing] a positive exclusion from all aspects of planning and contact with Health Authorities'. The CHC role in locality planning may be questioned, as may the need for such forums to arise at all, if CHCs were fully covering the ground. Even allowing for CHC interest to stretch far wider than joint working, their intermittent involvement again raises the whole question of the status and purpose of joint planning and working exercises.

The growing volume of practitioner literature on joint working is pointing to more experimentation, an increasingly central role for voluntary organizations side by side with health and social services, and perhaps paradoxically to practitioner awareness of the inevitably slow start and incremental approach which will characterize some of the 'best' joint working examples. Whilst accepting that 'lessons learnt' in one part of England may not translate easily to other settings, it is striking that attempts to summarize the 'learning' from particular instances, in terms of managerial approaches, and structural and procedural processes, are closely following one another. Thus, for example, Wright and Sheldon (1985) comparing joint working in one county council and one matching (now defunct) Area Health Authority, between 1979 and 1982, have highlighted factors which for them 'appeared crucial to efficient decisionmaking'. These included:

> the importance of personalities who can work well together, who are sufficiently high up in their authority to carry authority . . .
>
> clear, agreed operational guidelines between all services and members; tasks to be set/goals to be achieved . . .
>
> provision of an adequate data base from which to operate;
>
> and . . . time to allow relationships to develop to reach a point

where personnel are no longer defensive about their own services.

White (1988), analysing resource transfers taking place in 1985 and 1986 from North Lincolnshire Health Authority to Lincolnshire Social Services Department, emphasizes that 'mutual respect for each agency's motives, standards and independence is both a prerequisite and an outcome of collaboration'. McGrath's initial comments on the operation of the All-Wales Strategy includes reference to the need for commitment to the process, 'which is far more likely to develop where staff have been involved in the planning process'; and for some 'compromises in commitment to professional ideas . . . a willingness to understand the worlds others inhabit'. Stockton's conclusion, that there is 'no commonly recognised good joint project', identifies some generalized criteria for success, none of which are startlingly new, though some may need to be strongly emphasized for those who see joint working as simply a matter of 'getting liaison going' or its products as cheap service options (Stockton, 1988). These criteria include projects where

* philosophy and values are congruent;
* values are based on normalization for the consumer;
* and 'an entrepreneur is managing the process'.

In relation to the last criterion, Stockton envisages the 'engineers' of joint working, who 'know their machines intimately', though he falls short of identifying the particular disciplines and backgrounds from which such engineers might 'best' come. Much learning is clearly taking place as a result of joint working experiments, with each joint planning and working area having similar experiences.

Inevitably, ironies abound in relation to 'good' joint working, which may identify those local practices which are of limited value without the support of national policy developments. This may sound platitudinous, and be a source locally of much frustration. In North Staffordshire, for example, work on a joint strategy for disabled people has particularly highlighted serious shortfalls in staffing for occupational therapy, in both health and social services fields, and in physiotherapy and indicated a large unmet need for those services in the community. This situation is as much an issue of national training and remuneration policies in relation to these professionals as of local recruitment and retention problems in the

Potteries. The continuing issue of how to encourage and stimulate inter-professional working and mutual respect is so familiar in reports of joint working as to be highly unremarkable, yet at its base is the question of national policies on joint **training** for caring professionals, which is hardly high on individual professional groups' national agendas.

NEW LEADERSHIP FROM THE CENTRE?

With government policies for Community Care the major catalyst for joint working, and the new surge of ideas following the Griffiths Report on Community Care (DHSS, 1988), some of the 'old luxury' of joint working is ending, at the pace which local professionals would all accept and perhaps for only certain client groups. Certainly the predominance of health authorities as the 'lead' organizations in much joint working, through the joint planning and joint finance machinery, may be lessened. Whilst joint working would continue as centrally important, the Griffiths' report envisages an increased facilitating and enabling role for social services departments, and thus a shift in the power balance to those authorities, as joint finance allocation is transferred to them from the health authorities. One of the report's major concerns was the feasibility of establishing evident boundaries between a health service and a social service or social care responsibility, with the hope that the NHS and social services departments would be able to concentrate explicitly on 'health' and 'social care' needs respectively. Yet as Hunter and Judge (1988) in their critique of this report stress:

> The problem is of course that many individuals in the priority care groups, particularly elderly and physically handicapped people, move back and forth between health and social services, depending on their changing circumstances.

It is this complexity in people's lives which has given much of the rationale for the development joint working; and which is likely to defy any policy maker's attempt to ensure administrative convenience and tidiness. Hunter and Judge, looking to means for implementing in the face of these new challenges, feel that there may be scope for the creation of a semi-autonomous government agency, a Community Care Development Agency, with 'access to limited pump-priming funds to stimulate and facilitate innovative developments at local level'. The logic of this idea is that local equivalents might spring up to act as service providers for Community Care to straddle existing health and personal social service boundaries. This viewpoint was reached independently in North Staffordshire HA, where the notion of a Primary Care Authority has been mooted, for holding the 'community care' budgets for health, social services, grant in aid for voluntary bodies, and a proportion of Family Practitioner Committee funding, and distributing funds to any agency capable of delivering at set standards, given a competitive tender (Warren, 1989). Local 'care managers' would be appointed 'for instance . . . at local district council level', with populations around 80 000 – 90 000 – arguably close to the size of the Health Forums.

In such a radical option, separating the supplier of services from those setting standards and paying for the services, the primacy of the consumer might be seen to be paramount. What may be most in question will be sources of the entrepreneurs – or 'engineers' – with the ability as well as the commitment to manage such a new version of joint working (integrated rather collaborationist), with the 'old' joint working problems and a score of new ones. Once again, the issue is raised of the basis for and source of the particular types of managerial skills for experimental work which may become commonplace. It is tempting to speculate that for potential clients at least, there may be the preference that those managerial skills are to be found more in the health service than in social services departments, and that the expected Griffiths 'shift' towards ensuring social services departments take major lead responsibilities does not come about, because of the allegedly more acceptable status of being a client of the NHS as opposed to a client of the social services department. It is also possible that the delay in a governmental response to Griffiths' proposals reflected a patent unwillingness to increase elected local government responsibilities, as against those of the non-elected health authorities.

Joint planning and joint working futures, whether collaborational or partnership based, led by health or social services, are to an extent in the balance, whilst further decisions – or non-decisions – are reached on the feasibility of Griffiths' ideas. Community care policies may be the engine for ensuring its continuation, but the quality – and the quantity – of the products of the joint working engineers may be in some doubt. Internal structural reorganization

– or 'rationalization' – of statutory sector bodies is always a possibility, so that there can be no absolute certainties of the existing structural 'actors' remaining. The abolition of the English shire counties, and the transfer of services to the Districts, for example, has been a recent notion, mooted by, amongst others, the Association of District Councils. What effects, if any, the recent separation of the Health and Social Security elements of the former DHSS also remain to be seen.

The situation has been made vastly more complicated by the considerable variations in the policy ingredients for community care, as between the different components of the United Kingdom. If Wales 'leads', then Scotland may be thought to be 'laggardly'. Hunter and Wistow (1987a) emphasize the extent to which 'weaker variants of joint planning and joint finance were introduced in Scotland some years after they were in England and Wales', so that different parts of the Kingdom may be seen to reflect differing types of community care experiments and assumptions. In Northern Ireland, personal social services and health services are provided as an integrated service, through four Health and Social Services Boards.

Such differentials have been most recently highlighted in the government White Paper, Working for Patients (Department of Health, 1989b), where 'health promotion' receives mention only in relation to Wales. This is notable for its studied lack of reference to primary health care, the priority services and the future of community care management and funding. The frustration of many practitioners that these major omissions mean only 'part of the picture' for the future of health services (Jarrold, 1989) has been expressed widely, but some have identified in the 'blank sheet', opportunities for the community services, as well as leading hospitals, to become self-governing within an NHS framework. Such developments would undoubtedly attract and require the same type of entrepreneur that Stockton has identified as being vital for joint working success. The possibility for service fragmentation – an aspect of public service provision which arguably joint working is designed to defeat – appears to increase. Working Paper One, Self-Governing Hospitals (Department of Health, 1989a) outlines in one sentence the possibility of both greater independence for community health services, and thus their options to work with whom they choose, and greater division within the community health services, as these elements, across the country, do or do not seek self-government:

> it will often be sensible for a self-governing hospital to run a range of community-based services and indeed there might be a self-governing community unit.

The Griffiths report on community care points to the increasing importance of joint working, but with the power base for that work shifting from health and towards social services. With 'Working for Patients' proposing to remove local authorities' rights to nominate District Health Authority members, it seems increasingly unlikely that local authorities will become the dominant partner in community care work. This was perhaps further implied by the announcement in July 1990 of a postponement of major elements in the government's plans for community care. Nevertheless, the need for joint working continues, and it is possible that a stronger 'top-down' push for joint working will occur. Benson's typology of sources of change in promoting inter-organizational collaboration suggests the nature of the 'push', including firstly 'cooperative strategies' (where parties hold something of value for the other), secondly 'incentive strategies' (falling short of directives), and thirdly, 'authoritative strategies' (where organizations with common vertical ties are directed to engage in joint activities). (Benson, 1975). The All Wales Strategy may be seen as a partial example of the latter strategy, and a possible for model for future action, despite its limitations and shortcomings. Meanwhile, it seems likely that the managers and practitioners engaged in the tiring, demanding and unglamorous world of joint working are patiently committed to the longer term 'pay offs' which they are convinced such working will bring. How far patients are being patient with the results – or otherwise – of joint working is far less certain.

7

Satisfying the public and the consumer, or the public as consumer?

Allan McNaught

The problems and possible approaches to developing a 'consumer orientation' in community health services provides the focus of this chapter. Any critical observer of the NHS would find the current obsession with the 'consumer' rather fascinating, and requiring some explanation. The flowering of this concern is rather curious, given the legendary indifference of the NHS to the preferences and comforts of its consumers and established consumer champions. Who now, for example, remembers the humane recommendations and the non-implementation of the report on 'The pattern of the inpatient's day' (CHSC, 1961)? The characteristic NHS approach to consumer issues was recently restated by Taylor (1983), who observed that

> Where this [consumer surveys] has occurred it has been done on an ad-hoc basis either as a result of enlightened management or professional interests pressing to demonstrate inadequacy of existing services.

Contemporary concerns are somewhat different and their genesis can be traced to the Griffiths Inquiry into NHS management (DHSS, 1983). This report noted that

> Businessmen have a keen sense of how well they are looking after their customers. Whether the NHS is meeting the needs of the patients, and the community, and can prove that it is doing so, is open to question.

This positive articulation of the place of the consumer in health care raises concern with both the individual and the community and locates it in the heart of the organization, on the agenda of the new style general managers, causing

> district health authorities and general managers [to] move, of their own volition towards using market research techniques to inform their decision-making (Scrivens 1988, p. 177).

Most health journals now carry regular reports on particular consumer surveys, methodologies or attempts to improve the image or correspondence of a service to expressed consumer preferences. While not disagreeing with the proposition that the NHS needs to be more consumer sensitive, it is also important to be clear of its limits. In trying to give greater weight to consumer concerns, we need to acknowledge the wealth of organizational and political insights pertinent to this issue that already exists.

Three concepts are implicit in Griffiths' comments on the consumer: a definition of need; the needs of individual patients; and the needs of the community. This articulation is novel because it is directed at managers. Traditionally, the discourse on health needs has been almost the sole province of the medical and allied professions. This history, plus the existence of 'clinical freedom', means that management concern for consumer needs will probably always be somewhat circumscribed. Spencer's (1967) analysis and argument foreshadows current debate:

> It is clear therefore that everything that happens in a hospital under a HMC's [Hospital Management Committee] control is that Committee's responsibility. In practice the Committee can do no more than ensure that the junior doctors whom it appoints and the senior doctors who are appointed by the RHB [Regional Hospital Board] are suitably qualified and experienced . . . The satisfaction of the consumer's needs on the non-professional side is more directly within the management's control. (p. 132)

Spencer goes on to talk of the need to keep waiting times for outpatient appointments to the minimum, and how to ensure that waiting conditions are congenial. He even mentions a report on 'The reception and welfare of in-patients in hospitals' (CHSC, 1953), which gives advice which would hardly be out of place in 1989! However, it seems that for the NHS the needs of its consumer failed to be a major agenda item for managers until Griffiths forced it to their attention – a reflection of the predominant concern of service industries in the competitive 1980s.

This chapter will not examine the concept of need directly, but will take a sideways look at it through an exploration of the processes through which the NHS might develop greater sensitivity to individual and community needs, however, defined. Scrivens (1987) provides a useful definition that might assist us in this exploration. She draws a distinction between a 'consumer orientation' and 'consumerism'. The latter she defines as

> the organised efforts of consumers seeking redress, restitution and remedy for dissatisfaction they have accumulated in the acquisition of their standard of living (p. 20)

while a consumer orientation in service organizations

> means something more than just conducting market research or measuring whether services provided are acceptable. It means gearing up an organisation to espouse a set of values which permeate every strategic decision and which are present in every consumer contact . . . The organisation has to demonstrate this commitment, not only internally to its staff, but externally to the public, who have constantly to be reminded that the organisation is responding to the consumer interest. (p. 21)

This chapter will attempt to use Scriven's notion of 'consumer orientation' as a framework to assess and comment on current initiatives, particularly those based in community health services. Our starting point for this exploration will be the broader canvas: the community at large.

OLD WINE, OLD BOTTLES?

The traditional concern with health service consumers in aggregate has centred on public participation as a mechanism for accountability of the service to those who pay or benefit from its operations. The core issues here were about power, authority and accountability. The unwritten assumption was that if health providers were sufficiently accountable to users or if representatives of the public were an integral part of the decision-making process, then this would result in concern on the part of providers for the preferences and sensibilities of NHS users. These assumptions are reflected in Maxwell and Weaver's (1984) presentation of a variety of definitions and conceptions of public participation, as follows;

1. Consumer protection
2. Public consultation
3. Openess of managerial decision making
4. Full management participation by public representatives
5. Heightened individual and communal responsibility.

Until the establishment of Community Health Councils in 1976, participation in the NHS was not explicitly about consumer issues. The principal forms of participation that existed included Parliamentary debates and questions, and the appointment of local people and local authority councillors to health authorities and Family Practitioner Committees. In terms of their effect on health policy and day-to-day provision, these forms of representation and influence do not seem to have been very successful. Looking at Parliamentary influence on government [health] policy, Ingle and Tether (1981) argued that both Houses of Parliament were largely ineffectual in influencing the development of government policy at any stage of legislation' (p. 143) According to Ingle and Tether, Parliament was equally impotent in its day-to-day scrutiny of government business. Parliamentary questions, for example, 'were used to good effect' but were limited. Select Committees too were seen as largely ineffectual. Their diagnosis of the weakness of Parliament was not focused on its procedures or the poor support services available to the Houses or individual members. They saw the problem and the weakness as lying in the control of Parliament by political parties. For them members would only have influence over events

> if the hold on parliamentary procedures of partisan ideology is broken and this in turn will only happen as a consequence of the lessening of party discipline (Ingle and Tetler, 1981, p. 156).

There are problems, too, at the next level of public participation/accountability in NHS management. Health authority and Family Practitioner Committee members are appointed by and accountable to the Secretary of State. They are not elected nor are they delegates of some interest. In the words of HC (81) 6, all members

> are appointed to membership by the Secretary of State because

they are accountable to him for the discharge of their responsibilities. The Secretary of State is of course answerable to Parliament for the NHS as a whole.

In practice, members receive contradictory messages. While they
are accountable upwards, they are expected to behave as if local
needs and issues are their prime concern. A number of commentators and studies have suggested that health authority members
are not particularly effective (Hunter, 1981; Ham and Buchanan,
1985). Michael Spungin (1985), a member of Trent RHA, has
argued that the NHS is competently managed leaving 'no easily
discernible role for an amateur, part-time, inexperienced volunteer'.
He noted that options for major decisions have already been selec-
ted before they are presented to health authorities, leaving 'items
of little real importance' for members. Torkington (1983) is even
more forthright in her criticism of the lack of democratic or representative credentials of health authorities. She sees health authorities as being dominated by local political, professional and administrative representatives. As a result

> decisions which serve the interests of professionals and aca-
> demics are usually taken without any consultation with the local
> communities for whom resources are provided. (p. 20)

An interesting feature of this criticism is that Torkington does not
see local politicians as particularly representative. For Phillips
(1989), too

> The local community involvement on health authorities is very
> unsatisfactory: these people have been elected to **local** authorit-
> ies and then seconded to health authorities; moreover, they are
> all too well aware they are part of a hierarchial chain with their
> revenue controlled by national government.

This realization seems powerfully to shape the perception of members:

> Most of them chose to give the very broad general aim of making
> the best use of resources, deciding on the right priorities for
> the public/community and in a few cases, finding out what the
> public/community want and providing it. Those members whose
> aims were 'giving the public what they want' were all university
> or specialist medical representatives and did not, as might have

been expected, include the local authority nominees. (Day and Klein, 1987, p. 92)

In light of this finding, the proposal in the White Paper 'Working for Patients' (DHSS, 1989b) to 'depoliticize' the NHS by removing local councillors from health authorities seems rather curious. Day and Klein (1987), though, indicate a wider agenda in their observation that

> the process of producing technical tools of accountability needs to be 'politicised' if such tools are not to be seen as a threat or irrelevance by authority members. In other words the production of such tools should be seen for what it is: not just a neutral exercise in the application of objective expertise but as an argument about what should count as good performance. (p. 243)

It seems then that health authority members, whether one can call them representative or not, have a limited influence over the management of the NHS, the quality and style of services. Many writers have attributed this to the freedom which doctors enjoy from managerial control (Day and Klein, 1987; Elcock and Haywood, 1980). All, though, is not that simple. Day and Klein give this problem a new complication in their observation that:

> In short, the officers were seen as the monopolists of a particular kind of expertise, especially financial. And when members talked about the problems posed by professionalism in the NHS, they first and foremost were referring to the DMT (District Management Team) officers who, they sometimes felt, saw themselves dealing with intellectual challenges rather than providing a service. (p. 97)

Despite these problems, health authority members seem to exercise more influence than MPs, principally because they are nearer operational level, probably have a more limited agenda, and are able to marshal local social and political forces to influence decision making – but this has its limitations (McNaught, 1988, pp. 112–114).

What then of Community Health Councils – the so-called 'people's voice' in the NHS? Some 13 years after their creation most are not well known, even in their own local area. Most, too, seem to have only a marginal impact on NHS decision making. Scrivens

(1988) argues that their role is still uncertain, as they have been eclipsed by a number of developments including the introduction of general management, the new consumer orientation of health authorities (e.g. locality planning) and the growth of patients' participation groups in general practice. The Cumberlege Report on 'Neighbourhood Nursing' (DHSS, 1986a) suggested the establishment of local 'health care associations'. These were seen as a forum through which management and consumers could communicate and discuss service delivery and planning proposals. At the time, this suggestion was widely regarded as one which would further undermine the role of CHCs. However, these did not become a major initiative, although some 'locality planning' exercises seem to observe the same sort of process. Woodin (1985) reported on the experience of the community unit in Nottingham Health Authority of a consultation exercise organized by the local authority and voluntary organizations. This consultation exercise was part of a formal process to formulate proposal under Inner Areas Partnership. This consultation process consisted of two rounds of meetings held at 17 different locations in the city: 34 meetings in all. However, the apparent interest or concern of the public for health service issues was poor:

> In 1982, for instance, only four issues relating to health was raised . . . By 1984 there had been a limited increase [to six] . . . In 1985, however, there was a dramatic increase in matters being raised. (p. 1364)

The breakdown of issues raised is shown in Table 7.1.

Woodin saw a poorly informed public as the main reason for these results. The educational role of the meetings was seen as of great value and it is clear that there were some fairly fundamental gaps in public knowledge of the NHS:

> Lack of dentists, chemists and doctors was explained with reference to the status of these practitioners as independent contractors . . . Many members of the public were unhappy with this explanation and were clearly puzzled that a national service could exist on such privatised foundations. (p. 1365)

Taking an overview of developments and the balance of arguments it seems that we have all been the victims of sleight of hand: greater public accountability and public participation in the NHS is

Table 7.1. Issues raised at inner city consultation meetings, Nottingham

	Subject	*No. of times issue raised*
Health centres	(demand for, location, services required)	5
GP services	(more wanted, women GPs wanted, queries on 'emergency doctor' system)	5
Chiropody	(service wanted)	2
Dentist	(wanted)	1
Chemist	(more wanted, complaints about opening hours)	2
Mental illness	(information wanted)	3
Mental handicap	(facilities for)	2
Care in the community	(information wanted)	1
Health visitors	(information wanted)	1
Community health workers	(wanted)	1
A and E facilities	(wanted at additional location)	1
		24

Source: Woodin, J. 'Facing up to public opinion of the NHS', *Health and Social Service Journal*, October 31, 1985.

not the antithesis of greater sensitivity to the needs of the consumer. It seems, however, that the price which has been paid for greater consumer orientation is the loss of the vestiges of accountability and participation that existed, despite their short-comings. A consumer orientation in itself seems no guarantee of greater accountability, and may seem to be an apology for the reduction of accountability in the NHS:

One of the loudest sounds in contemporary public life is that of the buck being passed. Accountablity has been largely replaced by a refusal to take responsibility for things that go wrong. At the same time, the centralisation of so much policy making has meant that the public now has far less say over what is being done . . . Ministers are just too remote . . . What price local accountability in Exeter health authority, where 207 cancer patients received radiation overdoses last year at the Royal Devon and Exeter Hospital and where two physicists were sacked but where **no one** in the management hierarchy has resigned? (Phillips, 1989)

In considering 'consumer orientation' in the provision of CHS we are clearly dealing with a micro and macro problem. This section has looked at some of the more macro problems – the issues of accountability and participation in the decision-making and control process. Griffiths' notion of the community was rather simpler, and more passive. An aggregate of satisfied consumers seem to be his notion of the community. Robust strategies for CHS depend on consultation and collaboration between health authorities and a number of other statutory and voluntary agencies. Because there is no right or objective level of CHS provision this process of joint strategy development is rather more important and necessary for CHS than for hospital services. In Chapter Six Warren and Harrow show how difficult this is in practice, and that progress tends to be slow.

The proposed development of 'internal markets' for hospital services may make the process of hospital planning and development rather more obscure and secretive than it already is. Not so for CHS which will remain the responsibility of health authorities. The party political heat which is being generated over the 'internal market' proposal, and the intervening general election, before full implementation is likely to focus more attention on the NHS, particularly at local level. This again will, in my view, force the issue of accountability, participation and consultation with the broader public and/or its representatives – political, social, self appointed or otherwise – onto the health service agenda.

CONSUMERS IN A TOKEN ECONOMY?

Meeting the needs or aspirations of individual consumers or an aggregate of individual consumers is rather more discrete and manageable than that of the community or society at large. For the former a number of techniques or approaches are available – assuming that health service managers define this perspective as part of their job. However, we should not forget Spencer's (1969) comments on the limitations on management action as a result of clinical freedom and the professional culture of the NHS. Within these limits, it is quite clear that much more could be done to improve the presentation, organization and sensitivity of services, particularly in the way patients are handled by NHS staff (Rigge, 1985).

A good demonstration of what can be done by a motivated management is Goodwin's (1987) report of the 'patients are people' campaign at the Central Middlesex Hospital. With the advent of general management, the campaign was seen as

a useful adjunct to restructuring and redefining managerial responsibilities . . . [and] would help reaffirm the hospital's service oriented cultural values. (p. 248)

The Central Middlesex campaign was composed of three elements: (i) a staff training programme (with the help of the Industrial Society); (ii) publicity and patient involvement; and (iii) a variety of forms of staff involvement. A similar strategy is also reported by Ross (1985) for a hospital out-patient department. Reports on initiatives in community services have been rather thin. However, Haggard (1985) lists a number of ways of getting feedback from the public on community services. These include: suggestion boxes; patient/user groups; neighbourhood based local health service advisory groups; feedback surgeries (held by managers); surveys; lunch forums; maintaining a feedback file; more formal liaison with the community health council, and Quality Assurance manager; altering job descriptions of health centre administrators to include a feedback role; local consultation on plans; regular contact with voluntary bodies; annual grumble sessions for staff; informal small group consultative meetings; open meetings, etc.

A growing number of general practitioners are establishing 'Patients' Participation Groups', following Dr Peter Pritchard's example in Berinsfield in 1972. Most of these groups are instigated by doctors, and their usual reason for supporting these groups is that it enables them to be more sensitive to the needs and views of their patients. Many groups are associations of all practice patients, who elect a small committee to represent their interests. Some groups are much more informal and may just have a convenor/secretary. Some groups have developed their activities beyond that of being a voice and focus of interaction with the particular practice. Some undertake health education activities, community and practice support, fund raising, etc. Commonly, groups also provide an informal care service to other patients. This includes fetching prescriptions, evening and night-sitting, transport to surgeries, and so on. Several groups have also been successful in lobbying for improvements in local health and community services. However, most groups have problems in improving the level of participation by its potential members.

Both Haggard (1985) and Chambers (1987) see a consumer orientation as an integral part of health care delivery. Chambers also sees this as a source of countervailing power or an interest group that can be used to alter the outcome of decisions within the NHS (Chambers, 1987, p. 13). Rather naively, though, Chambers sees pursuing the interest of the consumer as conflict-free:

> In getting things right for the customer, managers can leave behind, for once, the no-win issue(s) . . . By contrast, the pursuit of the consumer viewpoint is relatively uncontroversial: it is difficult to deny the validity of the objective, and no specific service or function is under attack. (p. 13)

This conclusion defies both experience and commonsense. It also seems at odds with the case study of an attempt to improve Family Planning Services in Riverside Health Authority, reported in the same article by Chambers. Here signs of incipient conflict are evident:

> It has not been all plain sailing: some staff, particularly those originally employed by the Family Planning Association, have expressed some regret at the proposed shift in the function of the clinics, and have demonstrated some concern at the anticipated change in emphasis of their work. These worries will need to be more fully explored when the fuller programme to convert the service is known. (p. 14)

Another problematic issue is how one defines a consumer. If we take a mentally handicapped child, for example, who is the consumer? The child, its parents or both? And what are the implications of this for the conduct of a consumer-orientated strategy? Some of the problems and answers here can be read into Stuart Humphreys' work connected with the All-Wales Strategy for Mentally Handicapped People, in which he has described modes of parental participation in the planning of new services for the men-

tally handicapped. In his article Humphreys was concerned to dis-
cover the reasons for the non-response of the majority of parents
in the Vanguard area (of Gwynedd) to an invitatation to participate
in the planning of an integrated, locally based community service
for their district. A number of environmental and structural problems are highlighted as undermining parental participation. These
included a thinly scattered population, poor public transport, and
centrally based meetings held in the evening. His findings that
related to the characteristics of non-respondents were that:

- Some carers are sometimes so pre-occupied with their day-to-
  day tasks of caring that they do not have the time, energy or
  resources to enable them to participate.
- Many older carers have well established care routines that they
  have little desire to change.
- Parents who played an active role in voluntary or lobby groups
  at an earlier stage now believe that younger parents with more
  energy should respond.
- A small number of carers held the view that professionals have
  an uncaring attitude towards the mentally ill.
- Despite the publicity about the All-Wales Strategy, the majority
  of parents had only 'the vaguest idea' what the strategy was
  about.

Within the Vanguard area the level of parental participation
reached 30–40% at its peak and then steadily declined. In trying
to explain why this happened Humphreys looked closely at those
parents who participated in the consultative process. He classified
these participants as either 'Pragmatists', 'Democratic Radicals' or
'Patient Participators'. Pragmatists seek immediate, tangible benefits, 'with little cognisance of the complex organizational issues
local authority service providers had to contend with as a result of
the strategy'. This group became disenchanted and convinced that
administrators were ineffective – and disengaged from the process.
Democratic Radicals used the legitimate platform provided by the
Strategy to try to get 'apparently autonomous officers' within the
service-providing agencies to be more accountable to the wishes
of parents and the mentally handicapped. These are also seen as
moral crusaders and Humphreys details the discomfiture caused in
a 'Planning and Development Group' as:

Executive officers became trapped in a paradox. In order to deliver new services, frontline workers and administrators have to be appointed, but this move is interpreted as the setting up of a job creation fund. (p. 13)

Patient Participators were characterized by a 'wait and see' attitude towards information and concepts that they did not understand. This group went through a process of appreciation through which:

They begin to see things not just from the parental point of view ... They begin to enter more fully into the debate, not just as parents, who operate on the basis of particularistic knowledge, but as individuals who have travelled a difficult path with executive officers. They feel bona fide members of the planning group (p. 35)

The differences between these modes of participation are seen by Humphreys as the product of the preconceptions participants bring to the exercise. With Patient Participators, there is a predisposition towards collaboration which is facilitated by access to information and discussion, a degree of formal power and direct participation in the policy-making process. Pragmatists think participation should lead to quick improvements while

Radical democrats assume that the needs of the mentally handicapped will in the long run, be best served by the setting up of organisational structures which enable parents to make their views known and bring their ideas to fruition thus securing their rights and those of the mentally handicapped. (p. 35)

The work of Powell and Lovelock (1987) also shows that there can be multiple users/consumers of health services. They define consumers of a travelling day hospital (TDH) as:

the elderly people themselves, their relatives, and professionals outside the TDH team, but involved in the care and support of the particular group of patients who attend the TDH. (p. 17)

Powell and Lovelock saw the views and experiences of these users as

of great value in setting the content and quality of the service from the recipient's angle alongside questions of organisational style and its structural and other preconditions, discussions of which might become dangerously abstract, reflecting over-much the perspectives of professional carers, managers and planners. (p. 28)

For all this complexity, there are important questions and issues which a consumer-orientated approach can tackle, to the advantages of patients and the service alike. The note of caution struck by Lee (1986) should however serve to warn us of its limitations. He warned that 'market research is not a panacea' (p. 81).

CONCLUSIONS

At both the micro and macro level the notion of 'meeting the needs of consumers' can be either a passive or active process. At the macro level, consumerism has traditionally been a passive affair. The overwhelming objective has been to give consumer representatives some stake in the decision-making process. Within the particular environment in which the NHS has existed as a public service, the form of this participation has been more treasured than its content. The ideology surrounding this form of participation suggests that its benefits will 'trickle down' and result in a much more consumer sensitive service at the sharp end. The basic conclusion of this chapter is that the hopes for this form of participation have not materialized, whether at the macro or micro level. Despite this, the principle of participation at a macro level ought not to be jettisoned in a state that is becoming increasingly centralized.

The response of the NHS to the consumer/user at the micro level has, too, been rather passive. The recent Griffiths revolution and increasing concern with quality and the consumer have ushered in a more active conception of the consumer and their needs. A critical issue here is the extent to which consumer pressure or expressed needs falls outside the parameters set by managers and through what political or organizational processes managers bring some correspondence between the two. Scrivens (1988) has argued, for example, that the new consumerism of NHS management has pre-empted the role of the CHC. At a superficial level this is certainly true. However, it does leave CHCs ample room both to criticize district strategies and the quality of services provided, without ploughing the same furrow. Many CHCs have long criticized NHS management for its failure to be more responsive to the consumer/user of the NHS. The fact that the NHS is now trying to be more responsive, particularly at the micro level, has kicked off a redefinition of roles vis-à-vis CHCs and will lead to a rather messy process of both sides re-defining and re-learning certain aspects of their role and relationship.

With health districts, CHS seem a prime target for the new consumerism. It could be argued that as a largely ambulatory service, patient perception and the presentation of the service seem particularly important. Within this sector, health centres and clinics seem designed more for the convenience of health workers and planners, rather than for users. Examples of poor planning/presentation include child health clinics on first or second floors, with inadequate lift access – taking prams and disabilities into account – usually with no play space. Many new centres and clinics have rather inadequate and confused waiting and reception arrangements. In addition, despite the small size of many community premises many are in a fairly poor state of repair, so that in the professional press the up-grading of even small clinics is seen as some sort of management triumph (Shanks, 1984). A contrast can be drawn here with the modernization of optician's premises and the improvements in the quality of their services following the forced liberalization of optical services, much of which has passed without notice at 'street level' in the NHS. Clearly, much more needs to and can be done in CHS to improve the quality and presentation of services. The notion of the 'Health Care Shop' was floated in the 1986 White Paper (DHSS, 1986b), but it sank without a trace, while the much vaunted NHS review seems once again to have left CHS in a convenient backwater.

With community care the issues are rather more involved. The notion of 'normalization', the fact of multiple consumers, multiagency dependencies and the inability of many of the prime consumers to articulate their expectations leaves us with another set of paradoxes. Humphreys' (1987) work suggests that consumers/users who share the same world vision of service managers are more welcome than those who do not. This is not a surprising finding. However, given the sharp differences in aims and expectations in this field, managers should be wary of cultivating only those consumers with whom they feel comfortable.

What is clear from all this is that the public/consumer are not interchangeable concepts. The advances in consumer sensitivity are matched by other changes which seem to be making the NHS less accountable as an organization, to the public who are its paymasters. At the microlevel, the upsurge in consumerism seems to have countered what many saw as the creeping politicization of health care. The question, of course, is when consumerism has run its course, what then?

Part Three

Overview and Conclusions

8

Whither community health services? – harnessing the new public health and the new managerialism

Allan McNaught

Whilst an integral part of the NHS, the policy and management environment of CHS is marked by a need for negotiation, boundary management, clearer strategic and operational goals, and an improved public and professional image. At policy level, a variety of forces are at work which are rapidly changing the texture of the environment for CHS. In addition a range of new and more strident actors are entering the policy arena. Moore (1987), for example, has noted that:

> Slum housing, contaminated water and polluted air were some of the factors that prompted the first public health movement. Sadly more than a century later, these same issues are among the problems fuelling the second [public health] movement.

These threats to public health can be seen to have fairly direct consequences for personal health, and therefore for primary and community health services. These are highlighted by Player (1987a) in his report on one GP's experiences in Camberwell, South East London:

> Patients of mine are more and more people suffering from nervous breakdowns because of bad housing, because the backup from Social Services is not there or because they cannot get the [Social Security] benefits to which they are entitled.

Developing effective policies and programmes are obviously difficult in CHS because of the wide range of individuals, organizations and government agencies involved in primary and community health. This would be so even if some of the issues themselves were not horrendously complex or not marked by fairly deep clashes of interests. Some of these can be glimpsed in Player's (1987b) concern for the values and interests of our social and political leadership, and the machinations of those industries and interests whose activities, in his view, pose the contemporary threat to public health.

For Player our leadership seems to care little about the deprivations and suffering of ordinary people. At the same time, they seem to have been effectively courted and 'ear-stroked' by representatives or agents of these powerful interests.

At a macro-level it is clear the CHS policy making is intimately tied in with shifting social and political interests, expedience and ideologies. On this larger canvas it seems that health and welfare occupy a less prominent position in British social policy. The strident voice of the 'new public health movement' suggests that there have been some changes in the structure and commitment of a variety of groups, individuals and organizations to improving public health. However, this phenomenon can also be seen as an expression of the lower priority of health and welfare, with those who see themselves as welfare advocates arguing for more in a more hostile political environment.

Whatever one's conclusions about the socio-politics of public health, it is clear that something **is** happening, Harrow (Chapter One) and Dun (Chapter Five) provide evidence of increased local authority and voluntary sector initiatives and action in a segment of this policy arena. Although local authority initiatives have, to an extent, been driven by political considerations, their context and impact have been local, rather than national.

The spread of strategic management concepts and approaches in local government has, too, worked towards a more active local authority approach to health care. The work of Environmental Health and Social Services Departments has provided the organizational building blocks for this approach. Stimulus has also been given by the WHO 'Healthy Cities Programme', which also encouraged the creation of the 'Local Authority Health Network'.

At national level, government policy has been to exclude local authority representatives from District Health Authorities. This might lead to more adversarial relationships at local level; just when the organizational conditions for more fruitful collaboration and joint working may have been achieved in many health and local authorities for the first time since the 1974 NHS re-organization. The one hope is that increased local authority responsibility for community care of the mentally ill and handicapped, as envisaged in 'Caring for People' (HMSO, 1989), might provide a point of progressive contact with District Health Authorities.

The wide range of local authority and voluntary sector health initiatives, and forthright discussions of health issues are clear expressions of a changed CHS environment. They may also reflect an enhanced commitment and organizational capacity to tackle some of the more vexing health issues in local areas. However, the overall picture is one of complexity, conflict and surprise. That this should be so is not startling. What is welcome is the debate and the evident growing concern with the community's health.

These concerns are reflected at the management level of CHS. General and Unit management in the NHS have both created an organizational focus for community health issues. More curiously they have returned CHS to an organizational and management form resembling the old local authority health department, but in which the Unit General Manager replaces the Medical Officer of Health. This management structure and assumed processes provide hangers, on which the new concern for public health policy can be expressed at local level. Patch-based and locality management, within this structure provide a micro-focus for managers, health professionals, community activists and others.

These structures, processes and their potential alone are not able to address key questions about the nature of services and delivery strategies that are or should be followed in CHS. Kingsley and Douglas (Chapter 2) look at service strategies, using services for the mentally ill and handicapped as an example of some of the key issues. These are economically outlined in Figure 2.2. Here the actual design of services is only one element in the puzzle. But even this is not unproblematic as they argue that service design strategies also need to recognize the limits of our knowledge about what will be effective and to encompass the capacity to learn from failure. The manager is seen to have a key role in balancing external and internal forces around agreed service strategies. Like Player, Kingsley and Douglas see values as a key problem. They conceptualize the development of community care as a 'wicked' or moral problem, rather than a technical one. As such, the choices and processes are much more political than 'professional': 'a collaborative process for all the stakeholders to contribute to the choices which will have to be made' (p. 30).

The more technological under-pinnings of this process of choice are elegantly outlined by McArthur and Stone. They see better information and its utilization as necessary to the provision of better CHS. They advance a notion of a comprehensive information system, linking measures of need and how they are met with the availability of specific services and resources. Clearly this integration of information and its sensitive use will provide an objectively better basis for managerial action. However, history and experience suggests that technological developments/opportunities and managerial ideas will do not necessarily coincide, particularly in public sector management. In practice, we have to take into account some obvious and some rather subtle factors concerning managerial behaviour. Key here are the choices open to managers in what they do from day to day and the larger strategies they may or may not choose to pursue. Strategies for working with the voluntary sector (Chapter 5), local authorities (Chapter 6) and consumers (Chapter 7) all promote certain normative choices, and ones a manager need not accept or ones they can quite easily pursue without real commitment or conviction. Dun quite clearly saw these possibilities, when she noted that Unit General Managers might simply substitute management models for medical models making little difference to the communities they serve.

Further constraints on the choices open to UGMs and their possible responsiveness to these normative choices are envisaged by their short-term contract. However, Dun sees the value of UGMs courting Community Health Initiatives in order to create a more pluralist policy environment: a kind of balancing act between competing demands and cultures.

Warren and Harrow's argument for UGMs choosing to work more closely wth local authorities is much more managerial. They express a concern with 'Service fragmentation . . . efficiency and effectiveness' (p. 113). They assert that joint working needs to be 'managed' like any other health service initiative. Like Dun, they see fixed term contracts for UGMs as a possible barrier to more effective joint working.

McNaught welcomes the new emphasis on consumers, but sees problems in its practical implementation because of differences in interest, perception and the blurring of boundaries between customers/public participation. Community/public participation and consumer concerns run through the contributions by Dun, McNaught, and Warren and Harrow. The latter see the establishment of consumer/user participation across a wide spectrum at the 'pre-planning stage' as the most valuable and justifiable approach, although adding to the complexity of the management process. All this though has emphasized the centrality of personal, professional and organizational choices in CHS policy and management. Kingsley and Douglas's conception of strategy formulation in this field as a matter of moral or political choice leaves us with a rather inelegant and messy conclusion.

On the more positive side, it is clear that general and unit management offers a clearer organizational framework for choices, action and accountability. Clearly, too, locality or patch management offers a process and focus that is widely seen as right or appropriate for CHS and community care. This framework seems to make heterogeneous programmes, their goals and actual provision inescapable. What effort then should UGMs and planners expend to provide some coherent policy or strategic framework – and what should be its content? Kingsley and Douglas suggest that UGMs should be aiming at processes rather than goals.

> The ability to develop the capacity to generate new solutions and, through trying them, learning more about the development process and organization which could best deliver effective community services (p. 21).

Within CHS the possible solutions to service issues are rather wider than those typically available in acute hospital services, for example. Unlike acute services there are fewer guidelines and conventions about what shall be done and how. There are exceptions, however. The 'Better Services' documents have provided the foundation for current discussions and development in the care of the mentally ill and mentally handicapped. For the bulk of the CHS there is a considerable policy vacuum, which health authorities make policy 'on the hoof', and often in response to negative financial pressures. The current condition of health authority family planning services is a good example of a wider problem in CHS policy and management (Millar, 1987).

In the past a number of national reports have looked at particular policy areas in CHS. However, the lack of political commitment, the absence of general management in the NHS, and the poor quality of management in CHS and PHC has been a receipt for no progress. While these past documents provide useful background reading for new community UGMs they have their limitations. Their policy prescriptions need to be reassessed, as they were written for a particular policy and management agenda which may not be now relevant to CHS as a whole, or the circumstances of particular units.

More pointedly, Harrow and Dun have shown that the current CHS environment offers a host of new opportunities for tackling a series of 'wicked' problems. These could result in new initiatives and relationships with a better chance of success than single agency solutions – and might make moral choices easier, or less controversial.

General and unit management, and its technological accompaniments, offer an unrivalled opportunity to set the thinking, learning and action processes in motion. These can derive either particular or general answers to some of the questions about the role, direction and goals of CHS over the next decade.

Bibliography

Abrams, P. (1977) Community care – some research problems and priorities, *Policy and Politics*, **6**, 125–151.

Alaszewski, A., Tether, P. and Robinson, D. (1982) *Reorganisation of the National Health Service: Guidance for DHA members*, Institute for Health Studies, University of Hull.

Audit Commission (1986) *Making a Reality of Community Care*, HMSO, London.

Bachrach, L. (1980) Overview: model program for chronic mental patients, *American Journal of Psychology*, **137** (9), 1023–1031.

Barnes, J. and Bickler, G. (1987) *Southwark's Health: a Report on the Health of the Borough of Southwark*, Public Protection Department, London Borough of Southwark and Department of Community Medicine, King's College School of Medicine and Dentistry.

Baxter, C. (1987) Steps to sensitising the service, *Health Service Journal*, 4 June, 642–643.

Bayley, M., Parker, P., Seyd, R. and Tennant, A. (1987) *Practising Community Care: Developing locally-based practice*, Community Care: Social Services Monographs: Research in practice.

Bayliss, F. and Logan, P. (1987) *Primary Health Care for Homeless Single People in London: A Strategic Approach*, Working Party on Single Homelessness in London Health Sub-Group.

Beardshaw, V. (1987) The 'new' public health, *The Newsletter of the King's Fund*, **10** (3), Spring, np.

Beattie, A. (1985) Evaluating Community Health Initiatives – An overview, in Sommerville, G. *Community Development in Health: Addressing the Confusions*, King's Fund, London.

Benson, J. (1975) The inter-organisational network as a political economy, *Administrative Sciences Quarterly*, **20** (June), 229–250.

Bevan, A. (1952) *In Place of Fear*, Heinemann, London.

Black, D. (1980) 'Inequalities in Health'. Report of a research working party chaired by Sir Douglas Black, DHSS.

Bradshaw, J. (1972) Taxonomy of social needs, in McLachlan, G. (ed.)

Problems and Progress in Medical Care: Essays on Current Research
OUP, Oxford.
Brotherton, P. and Jenkins, J. (1988) Primary Lessons, *Newstatesman and Society*, 18 November, 15.
Bruce, N. (1981) *Teamwork for Preventive Care*, Research Studies Press, John Wiley and Sons Ltd., Chichester.
Bryson, J. (1988) Strategic planning: big wins and small wins, *Public Money and Management.* **8** (3), 11–16.
CACI (1986) CACI Updates – Small Area Population Estimates: 1986. CACI, London.
Catford, J. and Parish, R. (1988) *Heartbeat Wales in Action*, International Hospital Federation Yearbook, 1988, 130–132.
Central Health Service Council (CHSC) (1953) *The Reception and Welfare of In-patients in Hospital*, HMSO, London.
Central Health Service Council (CHSC): Standing Nursing Advisory Committee (1961) *The Pattern of the Inpatients' Day*, HMSO, London.
Chambers, N. (1987) Developing a consumer strategy in the NHS or getting things right, *Hospital and Health Services Review*, January, 12–14.
Chandler, J. A. (1988) *Public Policy-Making for Local Government*, Croom Helm, Beckenham, Kent.
Coalition for Community Care (CCC) (1988) Annual Report, 1988.
Collin, T. (1986) *Challenging Complacency in National Health Service Training: The report of an NHS Working group examining the strategic role planned training in managing*, Occasional Paper no. 3. NHSTA, Bristol.
Community Health Initiatives Resource Unit (CHIRU) (1987) *Guide to Community Projects*, National Community Health Resource, London.
Community Projects Foundation (1988) *Action for Health: Initiatives in Local Communities*, Community Projects Foundation, London.
Coobb, J. (1987) Bridging two worlds, *Community Outlook*, August, pp. 21–24.
Croft, S., Beresford, P. and Stanton, A. (1987) Consumers to the fore, *Community Care*, 26 November, 28–30.
Cumberlege, J. (1988) Medicine the Government may refuse to swallow, *Health Service Journal*, 24 March, 328.
Dalley, G. (1988) *Can 'Cumberlege' work in the inner city?* Working Paper for Managers, No. 4, Primary Health Care Group, King's Fund Centre, London.
Dalley, G. (1989a) *Patchworking – planning and managing primary health care in small areas.* unpublished report for the Department of Health, King's Fund Centre, London.
Dalley, G. (1989b) Professional ideology or organisational tribalism? The

health service-social work divide, in Taylor, R. and Ford, J. (eds) *Social Work and Health Care*, Research Highlights in Social Work, 19, Jessica Kingsley Publishers, London.

Dalley, G. and Brown, P. (1988) *Introducing neighbourhood nursing: the management of change*, Working Paper for Managers, No. 3, Primary Health Care Group, King's Fund Centre, London.

Dalley, G. and Shepherd, G. (1987) 'Going local' gathers speed, *Health Service Journal*, 23 July, 850–851.

Day, P. and Klein, R. (1987) *Accountabilities: Five public services*, Tavistock Publications, London.

Department of Health (1988) Circular (88) 64: Health Services Management: Health of the Population: Responsibilities of Health Authorities.

Department of Health (1989a) Annual reports on the health of the population, EL (89)P 1, January.

Department of Health (1989b) Working for patients, HMSO (Cmnd 555) London.

Department of Health (1989c) Working for patients. Working Paper 1, Self-Governing Hospitals 4

DHSS (1971) *Better services for the mentally handicapped*, HMSO (Cmnd 4683), London.

DHSS (1975) *Better services for the mentally ill*, HMSO (Cmnd 6233) London.

DHSS (1976) *Priorities for the health and personal social services*, HMSO, London.

DHSS/PSSC (1978) *Collaboration in community care: a discussion document*, HMSO, London.

DHSS (1979a) *Royal Commission on the NHS – report*, HMSO (Cmnd 7615), London.

DHSS (1979b) *Patients First*, HMSO, London.

DHSS (1980) Inequalities in health: Report of a research working party, DHSS, London (Chairman Sir Douglas Black).

DHSS (1983) NHS Management Inquiry, DHSS, London, DA(83) 38 (Chairman Sir Roy Griffiths).

DHSS (1984) Steering Group on Health Information: Fifth report to the Secretary of State, DHSS, London (Chairman Mrs Edith Korner).

DHSS (1985) Working Party on Disturbed Adolescents, DHSS, London.

DHSS (1986a) Neighbourhood nursing: A focus on care, DHSS, London (Chairman Mrs J. Cumberlege).

DHSS (1986b) Primary health care: An agenda for discussion, HMSO (Cmnd 9771), London.

DHSS (1987) Performance indicators for the NHS. Consultation Papers 1–9.

DHSS (1988) Community Care: An agenda for action, DHSS, London (Chairman Sir Roy Griffiths).

Dix, M., Moreton, W. and Jessop, E. (1987) Market research in the NHS: the Colchester health survey, Hospital and Health Services Review, January, 18–20.

Donaldson, I. (1986) Perception of patients' needs, Health Service Journal, 28 August, 1139.

Doyal, L. and Pennell, I. (1979) The Political Economy of Health, Pluto Press, London.

Drennan, V. (1985) Working in a different way: A research project examining community work methods and health visiting, Paddington and North Kensington Health Authority, London.

Drennan, V. (1986) Health visitors and homeless families, Health Visitor, **59**, 340–342.

Drennan, V. and Stearn, J. (1988) Health Visitors and Groups: Politics and Practice, Heinemann, London.

Dun, R. (1984) The relationship between occupational class and material deprivation. The experience of physical disability, University of Southampton, Faculty of Medicine, unpublished MSc. dissertation.

Dun R. (1987) Going local? A study of West Lambeth District Health Authority, unpublished report.

Dun, R. (1989) Pictures of health?, West Lambeth Health Authority, Community Unit.

Economist (1988) A slow cure for health, The Economist, London, 19 November, 37–38.

Elcock, H. and Haywood, S. (1980) The Buck Stops Where? Accountability and control in the National Health Service, Institute of Health Studies. Universty of Hull.

Elmore, R. (1982) Backward mapping: Implementation research and policy delusions, in Williams, W. (Ed.) Studying Implementation: Methodological and Administrative Issues, Chatham House, New Jersey.

Etherington, S. and Bosanquet, N. (1985) The Real Crisis in Community Care: Developing servicesfor mentally ill people, Campaign for the Mentally Handicapped, London.

Evans, J. K. (1981) Measurement and Management in Medicine and Health Services: Training needs and opportunities, The Rockefeller Foundation, New York.

Exeter and District CHC (1986) Locality planning – power to the people? A discussion paper.

Farrant, W. (1986) Health for all in inner cities: proposed framework for a community development approach to health promotion policy and planning at District level, Paddington and North Kensington CHC.

Faulkner, J. (1987) Transformation achieved by integration, *British Journal of Health Care Computing*, April 13–16.

Ferlie, E., Pahl, J. and Quine, L. (1984) Professional collaboration in services for mentally handicapped people, *Journal of Social Policy*, 185–202.

Forsyth, G. (1986) *Doctors and State Medicine: A study of the British health service*, Pitman Medical, London.

Fryer, P. (1987) Local Authorities and Health, in *Conference Report, Promoting Health in East Anglia*, 18 March 1987, East Anglia Regional Health Authority, 31.

Fryer, P. (1988) A Healthy City Strategy, three years on: the case of Oxford City Council, *Health Promotion*, **3** (2), 213–217.

Gaffeney, P. (1989) First steps taken to shape White Paper on care, *Community Care*, 20 July.

Gale, B., Garton, G. and Webster, A. (1988) The joint planning maze, in Stockford, D. *Integrating Care Systems: Practical perspectives*, Longman, London, pp. 1–13.

Glennerster, H. *et al.* (1983), *Planning for Priority Groups*, Martin Robertson, London.

Goldman, M. (1988) Britain pioneers putting patient notes on plastic, *Doctor*, 7 July, 20.

Goodwin, N. (1987) Implementing consumer awareness at unit level, *Hospital and Health Services Review*, November, 248–251.

Graessle, L. and Kingsley, S. (1986) *Measuring change, making changes*, National Community Health Resource, London.

Green, D. (1986) Joint finance: an analysis of the reasons for its limited success, *Policy and Politics*, **14** (2), 209–220.

Greenwood, R. (1987) Managerial Strategies in Local Government, *Public Administration*, **65** (3), 295–312.

Griffiths, R. (1983) Report of NHS Management Inquiry, published under cover of letter from Sir Roy Griffiths to the Secretary of State for Social Services, 6th October.

Griffiths, R. (1988) *Community Care: Agenda for Action*, HMSO, London.

Haggard, L. (1985) What do the patients say?' *Health and Social Service Journal*, 7 November, 1405.

Ham, C. (1986) Members in search of a role, *Health Service Journal*, 27 November, 1551.

Ham, C. and Buchanan, R. (1985) Health Authorities ill-prepared to make life and death judgements, *Health and Social Service Journal*, 21 March, 353–354.

Hambleton, R. and Hoggett, P. (eds) (1984) The Politics of Decentralisation: Theory and practice of a radical local government initiative. SAUS, Bristol University.

Harding, T. (1986) A stake in planning: joint planning and the voluntary sector. The community care project, National Council for Voluntary Organisations, London.

Harper, G. and Dobson, J. (1985) Participation: Report of a workshop involving people with mental handicaps and staff who work with them, campaign for the Mentally Handicapped, London.

Hatch, S. (1984) Participation in health, in Maxwell, R. and Weaver, N., *Public Participation in Health: Towards a Clearer View*, King's Fund, London.

Higgins, J. (1989) Defining Community Care, *Social Policy and Administration,* **23**, (1), May, 3–16.

HMSO (1957) *Royal Commission on the law relating to mental illness and mental deficiency*, HMSO, London.

HMSO (1985) Second Report from Social Service Select Committee. Session 1984–5, Community Care with special reference to adult mentally ill and mentally handicapped people [HC 13–i], HMSO, London.

HMSO (1986) *Primary health care: An agenda for discussion*, HMSO, London. Cmnd. 9771.

HMSO (1989) *Caring for People*, HMSO, London.

House of Commons (1985) Second Report from the social services select committee, session 1984–5, Community care: with special reference to adult mentally ill and mentally handicapped people, HMSO, London.

Hudson, B. (1987) Collaboration in social welfare: a framework for analysis, *Policy and Politics,* **15** (3), 175–182.

Hudson, B. (1988) Tried and tested in Wales, *Health Service Journal*, 26 May, 596.

Humphreys, S. (1987) Participation in practice, *Social Policy and Administration* **21** (1), 28–39.

Hunter, D. (1981) *Coping with Uncertainty: policy and politics in the NHS*, Research Studies Press, Chichester.

Hunter, D. and Judge, K. (1988) *Griffiths and Community Care: Meeting the challenge*, King's Fund, London.

Hunter, D. and Wistow, G. (1987) Community care in England, Scotland and Wales, *Public Money*, December, 27–30.

Hurst, M. and Stone, S. (1988) Information strategy for a community unit, *Health Services Management,* **84**, (5), 109–111.

IHSM (1984) *Hospital and Health Services Yearbook*, IHSM, London.

Ingle, S. and Tether, P. 1981 *Parliament and Health Policy, Gower, Aldershot.*

Jacobson, B. (1989) *Alliances for the New Public Health, Newsletter of the King's Fund*, June, **12** (2), np.

Jarman, B. (1983) Identification of underprivileged areas, *British Medical Journal,* **286**, 28 May, 1705–1708.

Jarrold, K. (1989) Prescription for health or recipe for disaster?, *Health Service Journal*, 9 February, 164.

Kershaw, G. (1987) Don't call us, *Health Service Journal*, 30 July, 883.

King, D. (1986) The local dimension: care in the community, in Parston, G. (ed.) *Manager as Strategist: Health service managers reflecting on practice*, King's Fund, London.

Kings Fund Centre (1982) *An Ordinary Life: comprehensive locally based residential services for mentally handicapped people*, Project Paper No 24, London, King Edward's Hospital Fund for London.

Kings Fund Centre (1984), *An Ordinary Working Life (Vocational Services for People with Mental Handicap)* Project Paper No 50, London, King Edward's Hospital Fund for London.

Kings Fund (1987a), *Living Well into Old Age*, London, King Edward's Hospital Fund for London.

King's Fund Centre (1987b) *Patching In – a newsletter for managers, 2*, King's Fund Centre, London.

King's Fund Centre (1987c) *Decentralising community health services – report of a conference*, King's Fund Centre, London.

Kingsley, S. and Smith, H. (1989) *Values for a Change*, King Edward's Hospital Fund for London, London.

Kingsley, S. and Towell, D. (1988) Planning for High Quality Local Services, in A. Lavender and F. Holloway (eds) *Community Care in Practice: Services for the Continuing Care Client*, John Wiley and Sons, Chichester.

Klein, R. (1983) *The Politics of the National Health Service*, Longman, London.

Kohn, R. (1977) *Coordinating health and welfare services in four countries: Austria, Italy, Poland and Sweden*, WHO, European Office, Copenhagen.

Lee, R. (1986) Market research for health authorities, *Hospital and Health Services Review*. March, 79–81.

Levitt, R. (1976) *The Reorganised National Health Service*, Croom Helm, London.

London Health Planning Consortium (1981) Primary health care in inner London: report of a study group [Acheson Report], DHSS, London.

Long, C. and Bourne, V. (1987) Linking professional and self-help resources for anxiety management: community project, *Journal of the Royal College of General Practitioners*, May, 199–201.

Lulham, S. (1988) Management data from patient care, *British Journal of Healthcare Computing*, April, 13–16.

McGarth, M. (1988) Inter-agency collaboration in the All-Wales Strategy: Initial comments on a Vanguard Area, *Social Policy and Administration*, **22** (1), 53–67.

McKeganey, N. and Hunter, D. (1986) 'Only connect . . .': tightrope walking and joint working in the care of the elderly, *Policy and Politics*, **14** (3), 335–360.

McNaught, A. (1987) *Health Action and Ethnic Minorities*, Bedford Square Press, London [for National Community Health Resource].

McNaught, A. (1988) *Race and Health Policy*, Croom Helm, London.

Maher, J. and Russell, O. (1988) Serving People with very challenging behaviour, in D. Towell (ed.) *An Ordinary Life in Practice: Developing comprehensive community based services for people with learning disabilities*, King Edward's Hospital Fund for London, London.

Malin, N. (1987) Principles, Policy and Practice, in N. Malin (ed.) *Reassessing Community Care*, Croom Helm, London.

Mansell, J. (1988) Training for Service Development', in D. Towell (ed.) *An Ordinary Life in Practice: Developing comprehensive community based services for people with learning disablities*, King Edward's Hospital Fund for London, London.

Martin, J. P. (1984) *Hospitals in Trouble*, Blackwell, Oxford.

Maxwell, R. J. (1984) Quality assessment in health, *British Medical Journal*, **288** 6428.

Maxwell, R. (ed.) (1988) *Reshaping the National Health Service*, Policy Journals, Hermitage, Berkshire.

Maxwell, R. and Weaver, N. (eds) (1984) *Public participation in health: Towards a clearer view*, King's Fund, London.

Millar, B. (1987) NHS Family Planning – will it fade away? *Health Service Journal*, Sept. 24, 1099.

Ministry of Health (1965) *Report of the Committee on Local Authority and allied personal social service*, HMSO, London.

Moore, W. Building a public health alliance, *Health Service Journal*, July 23, 1987, 842–843.

Morley, M. (1987) Policy Making for Ill-health Prevention; the local authority role in ill-health prevention, *Local Government Policy Making*, **14** (1), June, 50.

Morris, R. (1984) The challenge to health planning and provision, 45–53, in Sommerville, G. (ed.) *Community Developments in Health: Addressing the Confusions*, Kings Fund, London.

National Association of Health Authorities [NAHA] and National Council Voluntary Organisations (NCVO) (1987) *Partnership for Health*, NAHA, Birmingham.

National Community Health Resource (1988) *A New Voice for Health*, NCHR, London.

National Health Service Training Authority (NHSTA) (1986) *Services for people with mental handicap: Human resource issues*, NHSTA, Paper No. 2.

National Institute for Social Work (1982) *Social workers: their role and tasks*, [Barclay Report] Bedford Square Press/NISW, London.

NCVO Community Care Project (1987) *Practice notes: Developing voluntary sector partcipation in joint planning*, NCVO Community Care Project, London.

Nightingale, S. (1988) Joint Planning: Unremarkable but productive, Health Services Management, August, 76–79.

Nocon, A. (1989) Forms of ignorance and their role in the joint planning process, *Social Policy and Administration*, **23** (1), 31–47.

O'Brien, J. (1987) Embracing Ignorance, Error and Fallibility: Competencies for leadership of effective services, in S. Taylor (ed.) *Community Integration*, N. Y. Teachers College Press of Columbia University, Columbia, New York.

Office of Population Census and Surveys (OPCS) *OPCS Newsletter to the NHS* [Issued quarterly] OPCS, Hampshire.

Pahl, J. and Vaile, M. (1988) Health and health care among travellers, *Journal of Social Policy*, **17** (2), 195–213.

Parston, G. (1980) *Planners, Politics and Health Services*, Croom Helm, London.

Parston, G. (1986) Learning to use plans and guidelines, in G. Parston (ed.) *Managers as Strategists: Health services managers reflecting on practice*, King Edward's Hospital Fund for London, London.

Phillips, M. (1989) There's no accounting for national health, *The Guardian*, 6 January, 21.

Player, D. (1987a) Civilised chat that allows the killing to continue, *Health Service Journal*, 23 July, 853.

Player, D. (1987b) Deprived of caring leaders, *Health Service Journal*, 20 August 963.

Portwood, D. (1986) Local authorities unemployment strategies, *Social Policy and Administration*, **20** (3), Autumn, 217–224.

Powell, J. and Lovelock, R. (1987) The role of consumers' views in the evaluation of services: A case study – the travelling day hospital, *Social Services Research*, No. 1, 16–29.

Price, L. (1989) Evaluation at the Wells Park Health Project, *Community Health Action*, No 12, Spring, 13.

Prowse, M. (1988) A new dependence on charity, *Financial Times*, 31 October, 16.

Ramon, S. and Giannichedda, M. (eds) (1988) *Psychiatry in Transition: The British and Italian Experiences*, Pluto Press, London.

Rathwell, T. (1987) *Strategic Planning in the Health Sector*, Croom Helm, London.

Rigge, M. (1985) The customer's perspective in Consumerism in the NHS, *Health and Social Service Journal*, Centre Eight, 30 May, 4–5.

Rittel, H. W. J. and Weber, M. M. (1974) Dilemmas in a general theory of planning, in R. L. Ackoff (ed.) *Systems and Management Annual 1974*, New York, Petrocelli; reprinted in F. E. Emery (ed.) (1981), *Systems Thinking* Vol. 2. Penguin, Harmondsworth.

Rosenthal, H. (1983) Neighbourhood health projects: some new approaches to health and community work in parts of the United Kingdom, *Community Development Journal* **18** (2), 120–131.

Ross, P. (1985) quoted in Deer, B. and Rayment, T. NHS team set for purge on doctors, *Sunday Times*, 17 March.

Scott-Samuel, A. (1989) The new public health: Speke Neighbourhood Health Group, in Seedhouse, D. and Cribb, A. (eds) *Changing Ideas in Health Care*, John Wiley, New York.

Scrivens, E. (1987) Developing a consumer orientation in the NHS, *Health Care Management*, **1** (3) 19–23.

Scrivens, E. (1988) Consumers' accountability and quality of service, in Maxwell, R (1988) *Reshaping the National Health Service*, Policy Journals, Hermitage.

Shanks, T. (1984) A clinic under seige, *Hospital and Health Services Review*, March, 75–77.

Sherman, J. (1989) Local authorities to look after the old and the mentally ill, *The Times*, 13 July, 5.

Smith, A. (1988) The nation's health: a strategy for the 1990s. A report of an independent multi-disciplinary committee chaired by Professor A. Smith, King's Fund.

Somerville, G. (1985) Community Development in Health: Addressing the Confusions, King's Fund, London.

Spencer, J. (1967) *Management in Hospitals*, Faber and Faber, London.

Spungin, M. (1985) 'Excuse my ignorance but what am I doing here?', *Health and Social Service Journal*, 20 June, 765.

Standing Medical Advisory Committee and Standing Nursing and Midwifery Advisory Committee (1981) *The primary health care team*, [Harding Report]HMSO, London.

Stewart, J. (1985) *Strategic management in local government: A discusson paper*, Local Government Training Board, London.

Stewart, J. D. (1986) *The New Management of Local Government*, Allen and Unwin, London.

Stocking, B. (1985) *Initiative and inertia: case studies in the NHS*, Nuffield Provincial Hospital Trust, Oxford.

Stockton, D. (ed.) (1988) *Integrating Care Systems: Practical perspectives*, Longman, London.

Strong, P. (1988) The impact of general management on the NHS, *Radical Community Medicine*, **34**, Summer, 51–53.

Taylor, M. (1983) The NHS and the consumer, *Hospital and Health Services Review*, July, 176–180.

Thomson, E. C. G. (undated), Slough Borough Council Health Strategy statement.

Timmins, N. (1990) Changes in community care to be postponed, *The Independent*, 9 July, 1.

Torkington, P. (1983) The racial politics of health: A Liverpool profile, Merseyside Area Profile Group. University of Liverpool.

Towell, D. (ed.) (1988) *An Ordinary Life in Practice: Developing comprehensive community based services for people with learning disabilities*, King Edward's Hospital Fund for London, London.

Towell, D. and Kingsley, S. (1988) Changing Psychiatric Services in Britain, in S. Ramon and M. Giannichedda (eds), *Psychiatry in Transition: The British and Italian Experiences*, Pluto Press, London.

Tyne, A. and O'Brien, J. (1981) *The Principle of Normalisation: A Foundation for effective services*, CMH Publications, London.

Walker, A. and Townsend, P. (eds) (1981) *Disability in Britain. A manifesto of rights*, Martin Robertson, Oxford.

Warren, G. (1987) Introducing decentralisation and participation within a community unit, MSc dissertation, CNAA, London.

Warren, G. (1989) Primary Care Authority, unpublished.

Watt, A. (1984) Community health initiatives: Clarifying the complexities within the community health movement. Paper given at King's Fund Centre conference.

Welsh Office (1983) *All-Wales strategy for the development of services for mentally handicapped people*, Welsh Office, Cardiff.

Welton, J. and Evans, J. (1986) The development and implementation of special education policy; where did the 1981 Act fit in? *Public Administration*, **64** (2), 209–227.

White, M. (1988) Negotiating resource transfers, in D. Stockton, *Integrating Care Systems: Practical perspectives*, Longman, London.

Whitehead, M. (1987) *The Health Divide*, Health Education Council.

Wilce, G. (1988) *A Place Like Home: A radical experiment in health care*, Bedford Square Press, London.

Wolfensberger, W. (1972) *The Principle of Normalisation in Human Services*, NIMR, Toronto.

Woodin, J. (1985) Facing up to public opinion of the NHS, *Health and Social Service Journal*, 31 October, 1364–1365.

Wright, J. and Sheldon, F. (1985) Health and social services planning, *Social Policy and Administration*, **19** (3), 258–271.

Index